# A HOLISTIC APPROACH TO UNDERSTANDING AND TREATING COMMON MEDICAL PROBLEMS

HANDBOOK OF COMMON
MEDICAL PROBLEMS

# A HOLISTIC APPROACH TO UNDERSTANDING AND TREATING COMMON MEDICAL PROBLEMS

Dr. Sanjay Srivatsa, MD FACC
Medical Director
Institute of Healthy Living

Katarzyna Dorosz
Institute of Longevity

Cover photo: Maarten Van Dijk, Beata Izabela Jastrzębska
DTP: Alfa Skład Łukasz Bieszke

All rights reserved, no part of this book can be published not reproduced in any form without the written permission of the publisher.

*We dedicate this book
with gratitude to our beloved Parents*

*Raghu and Meera Srivatsa*

# Table of Contents

**INTRODUCTION** ......................................................................... 9

**Chapter 1** The Heart ..................................................................11
**Chapter 2** Diabetes ................................................................ 117
**Chapter 3** Varicose veins ..................................................... 167
**Chapter 4** Cholesterol ........................................................... 201
**Chapter 5** Healthy heart and stress ................................... 227
**Chapter 6** Prostate ................................................................ 243

# INTRODUCTION

In this book, we have attempted to present **everyday medical problems** in a simple, and scientifically accurate style, but avoiding confusing or overly technical jargon to make it easily accessible to the general public. Today, with the availability of the internet everywhere, copious information is readily available regarding many medical conditions in an instantaneous manner. However, this information is cumbersome in nature, being more encyclopedic than concise, or practically helpful to the ordinary reader. This compendium takes a more pragmatic and focused approach to informing its readers. We have aimed to be **selective** in our approach. Here, we present several common medical conditions starting with their causation and symptoms, then outlining suitable therapy and finally complimenting this with **holistic pragmatic advice** on the day to day management of these problems. While avoiding a cookbook approach, our emphasis has been throughout to help the reader help themselves (or their family members) with sound medical advice based on established scientific principles, complimented by practical advice on the use of readily available herbs, nutritional supplements, exercise, and relaxation therapies. We have included **specific recommendations on diet, physical activity, medications, and complimentary approaches** including exercise, meditation, yoga, as well as numerous other important health enhancing lifestyle strategies.

Our hope is that the reader will use this book as an "easy read" **go to reference** to regularly look up medical diseases and disorders, in order to facilitate understanding and management of their own medical conditions. To this end, we have created a book that is up to date with both the scientific mechanism of disease as well as state of the art medical treatments both allopathic and alternative.

We believe informed discussion between our readers, augmented by the assistance and direction of their own personal physicians is the best approach to health maintenance. A word of caution: if using herbs and other supplements as adjuncts to therapy, please be sure to consult with your physician, to ensure there are no interactions with prescribed medications or other contraindications. All other suggestions made by the authors are fully compatible with conventional medical approaches throughout the world. Finally, we would welcome suggestions and comments to improve and expand our handy reference book, so together we can enhance the welfare and wellbeing of all those who read this book.

With every wish for the health
and happiness of our readers,
**S. Sanjay Srivatsa MD FACC FACP**
**Katarzyna Dorosz**

INSTITUTE FOR HEALTHY
LIVING CALIFORNIA USA

# Chapter 1
# The Heart

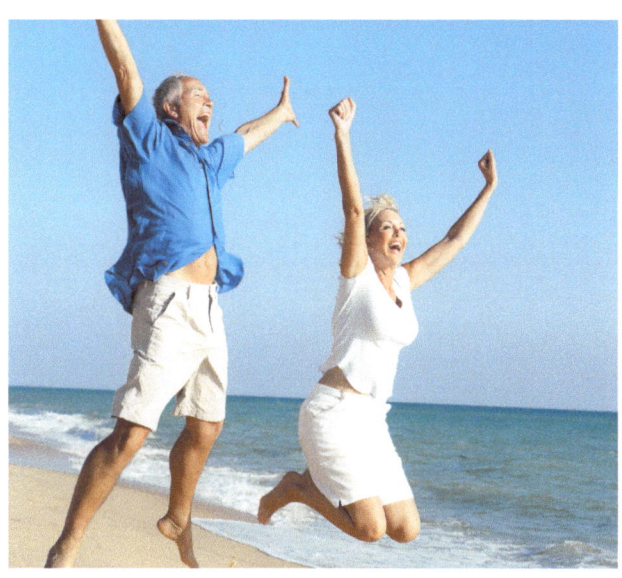

The heart is a muscular organ that pumps blood throughout the body. It is in the middle cavity of the chest, between the lungs. In most people, the heart is located on the left side of the chest, beneath the breastbone (though in rare cases it can reside on the right side of the chest).

The heart is composed of smooth muscle. It has four chambers which contract in a specific order, allowing the human heart to pump blood from the body to the lungs and back again with high efficiency. The heart also contains "pacemaker" cells in a region called the sinoatrial node, which fire nerve impulses at regular intervals, which when conducted down the heart's conduction system (called the HisPurkinje fibers) stimulate the heart muscle to contract.

**Heart**

This graphic shows the functioning of this extraordinarily complex pump in action. The heart is one of the most vital and delicate organs in the body. If it does not function properly, all other organs – including the brain – begin to die from lack of oxygen within just a few minutes. As of 2009, the most common cause of death in the world was **heart disease.**

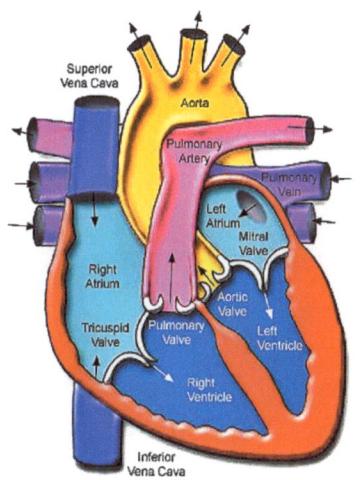

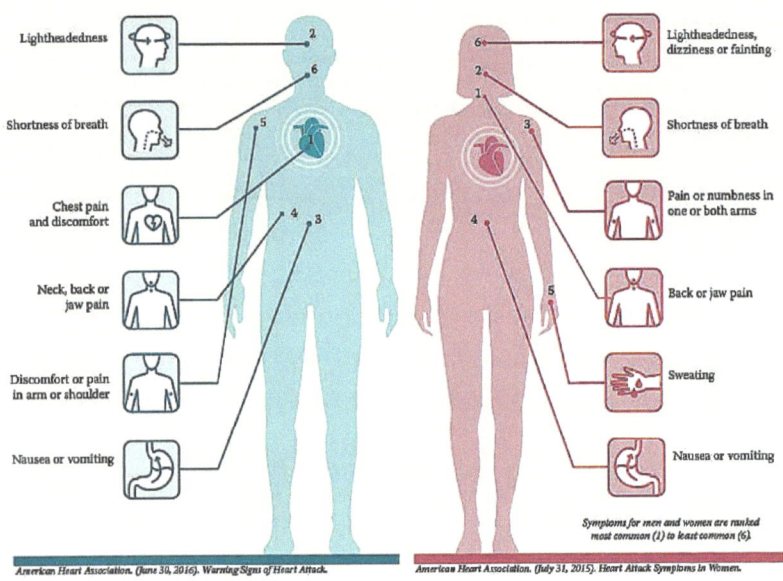

Most heart disease occurs because of advancing age or lifestyle. As a person gets older, cholesterol can build up in the arteries, a process called **"atherosclerosis",** and this is more likely for people who have diets high in saturated fat and cholesterol. Rarely, however, heart disease can also occur due to a viral or bacterial infection of the heart or its protective tissues.

Scientists have had some success replicating the heart's pumping action with artificial pumps, but these pumps can be rejected by the body, and they break down over time, from mechanical wear and tear.

**Cardiology** is the field of study that includes both the heart and the vascular system. Today, the astute realization that the heart and vascular systems are not only anatomically and physiologically innately the same, has led to a greater emphasis on vascular care. One impetus to this movement towards vascular care has been the rise in obesity, diabetes and the consequential rise in hypertension (high blood pressure), adverse lipid levels, and metabolic changes which maintained long term has led to a rise in the prevalence of myocardial infarction (heart attacks), strokes, heart failure and kidney disease. These consequences can be prevented with a little individual and societal effort. It is ironic to note that while starvation, poverty, and infectious disease ravages some parts of the world, the scourge of industrial nations appears to be a surfeit of the worst things for cardiovascular health namely smoking, alcohol, salt, greasy food, and sedentary behavior. We have taken the old phrase "eat, drink, and be merry" to heart literally as cardiovascular risk has risen to new levels across the world. So, cardiology lies at the nexus of many ailments and the careful attention to genetic risks, environmental issues (especially pollution), and human behavior is part and parcel of preventative medicine today. Cardiologists would much rather be ardent preachers of preventative care, than healers of inevitable disease.

## How big is the scale of the problems associated with heart disease?

The scale of the problem is daunting but not insurmountable. Cardiovascular disease (CVD) today is responsible for approximately **onethird of all deaths worldwide,** is steadily increasing in both developing and developed countries as the prevalence of risk factors for cardiovascular disease relentlessly increases: dyslipidemia, hypertension, obesity, diabetes, physical inactivity, poor diet, and smoking. Although these are modifiable risk factors, measures to prevent or control them, particularly in developing countries are in their earliest phases. A population based strategy for CVD prevention in high risk populations, could greatly reduce the burden of future cardiovascular disease. The ravages of CVD if modifiable risk factors are left unchecked in the coming decades will be staggering. This will take both courage and initiative on an individual and statewide basis across all ethnicities, in almost all major populations across the world to achieve.

**Cardiovascular disease (CVD)** is a major health problem across the world, accounting for 30% of all deaths. Of the 58 million deaths from all causes worldwide in 2005, an estimated 17.5 million were due to CVD, 3 times more deaths than are caused by infectious diseases including HIV/AIDS, tuberculosis, and malaria combined. It is estimated that non – communicable conditions will account for more than three – fourths of all deaths in 2030, and deaths from CVD will rise to 23.4 million, an approximately 37% increase from 2004 rates. Furthermore, the leading causes of death in the world in 2030 are predicted to be ischemic heart disease (IHD) and cerebrovascular disease (stroke), which together account for the majority of CVD.

The **World Health Organization (WHO)** points out that CVD has no geographic, socioeconomic, or gender boundaries. CVD is the leading cause of death in developing as well as developed countries.

Both low and middleincome countries contribute to about 80% of CVD deaths. Stroke deaths in low and middleincome countries are 5 times more likely than in highincome countries. In developed countries, lower socioeconomic groups have a higher prevalence of risk factors, higher incidence of disease, and higher mortality. As the **CVD epidemic** escalates in developing countries, the greatest disease burden will shift to lower socioeconomic groups. Among women across the world, heart disease is the also the most common cause of death. Although CVD is the leading cause of death for women as well as men, women are generally a decade older than men when CVD develops. Since 1949 when the seminal Framingham Heart Study was initiated, it was realized that cardiac health can be influenced by lifestyle and environmental factors, and by inheritance. The **9 simple risk factors** that predict CVD are abnormal lipids, hypertension (high blood pressure), smoking (also vaping), diabetes, abdominal obesity, physical inactivity, unhealthy diet, excessive alcohol consumption, and psychosocial stress. In addition, in developed and developing countries, low income and poor education status have been consistently associated with increased CVD mortality and higher rates of CVD risk factors e.g. smoking, obesity, and hypertension. It was not until recently in 2004 that the **INTERHEART** study, which studied over 15,000 cases of acute myocardial infarction (heart attack) in 52 countries across the world pointed out that **over 90% of all the risk could be predicted by these 9 risk factors**. In the INTERHEART study, twothirds of women with AMI were 60 years or older, compared with 40% of men. Smoking as a cause death from CVD (and lung cancer) has been scientifically established since the 1950's. It has taken the better part of over half a century, to establish governmental policies that populationbased health care behavior that promotes the cardiovascular health and longevity of all populations across the world. The rise of obesity, inactivity, diabetes, hypertension and smoking in men and women in developing nations and low economic status populations, has fueled an alarming rise in CVD prevalence. So that while death from CVD has declined as an absolute percentage rate in developed countries such as the USA and Europe, the reverse is true in developing countries including Central / East European and South East Asian countries. The mean age for the first presentation of AMI in Africa, the Middle East, and South Asia was ten years younger compared with other regions of the world. This predicts a large increase in cardiovascular disease in these regions in the forthcoming years.

**Two key findings** were found in the **INTERHEART** study. The **first key finding** is that, wherever you look, in every society, there is a **very strong and causal association between smoking and cardiovascular disease**. While not a new revelation this finding was a very strong correlation across all populations and is particularly striking in developing countries, urbanized populations, and lowincome socioeconomic groups. **INTERHEART showed that smoking 15 cigarettes daily increases the risk of a heart attack by 40%.** This could cancel the beneficial effects of other secondary preventions, such as aspirin, which reduces risk by 20%; it could also eliminate as much as 75% of the benefit of taking a statin.

This risk increases with the amount of tobacco smoked per day (OR 9.2 and in those who smoke>40 cigarettes per day). **All forms of tobacco, including filtered and nonfiltered cigarettes, electronic cigarettes, vaping, pipes and cigars, and chewing tobacco, are harmful.**

This is the basis for the call by many health care providers for effective governmental policy across the world to **reduce and eliminate smoking entirely** using education, taxation, banning of smoking in public areas, and formal smoking cessation programs etc. Electronic cigarettes whose use in vaping especially by teenagers is fueling a new wave of cardiovascular risk. ecigarette, or vaping, product use can cause lung injury (**EVALI**). Lung damage is caused by inhaling viscous oils, sometimes added as thickening agents to blackmarket vaping products, especially to THCvaping cartridges. One such oil is called vitamin E acetate, and it was found in many — but not all — of the product samples from patients, which were recently tested by federal officials. Of the 225 THCcontaining products tested, 47% contained vitamin E acetate. This issue has resulted in banning these vaping products for public safety reasons by many state and federal governments.

The **second key finding** is that psychosocial risk factors, including **stress, anxiety, depression and low generalized feelings of control, were responsible for 32.5% of the population attributable risk for heart attacks**. This is remarkable given that the populationbased risk attributable to smoking was 35% and that for obesity (20%) and hypertension (18%). It suggests that we have considerable opportunity in **altering lifestyle** to not only increase aerobic physical activity, modify diet, prevent smoking, control blood pressure, treat or prevent diabetes, but also to **treat stress, anxiety, or depression.**

Every physician extrapolates populationbased risk factor analysis to the treatment of individual patients. Many patients undergo physical checkups and laboratory testing as well as stress tests to discover and treat coronary and vascular disease before CVD becomes overtly symptomatic. **Newer noninvasive imaging techniques such as cardiac/coronary CT and cardiac MRI can demonstrate disease before symptoms are evident.** The challenge has been to modify the environmental and individual CVD risk factors to alter or prevent future adverse outcomes in such patients. It sounds like 20/20 hindsight to say it, but an ounce of prevention is worth a pound of cure, and the best opportunity for prevention, is altering risky behavior in childhood. The educational, political, and social impetus to achieve such an undeniably desirable outcome is still lacking everywhere around the world. The rise in morbid obesity and diabetes in children in developing and developed countries is a sobering testament to the failure of our individual and political resolution to prevent CVD death in these children at later ages. The future does not bode well if our governments and educational systems do not act and soon. Universal affordable health care would be a big step in the right direction.

**Is heart disease hereditary?**
**How can we help raise awareness?**

A strong hereditary component exists for cardiovascular disease (CVD) both atherosclerotic diseases of the coronary artery (coronary artery obstructive disease from atheromatous plaque), arrhythmias (electrical abnormalities of conduction system of the heart) and myocardial disease (cardiac muscle diseases). The interplay of genetics and environment is always at the forefront of disease outcomes, and so it is with cardiovascular disease. The human heritability of CAD is estimated to be between **30% and 60%**. Only 10% of human CAD variation is currently explained by the known CVD risk genes, i.e. CVD genetic risk is explained by mostly novel loci that have not yet been investigated. Despite the complete sequencing of the human genome, the complexity of interaction between multiple cardiovascular disease gene loci is daunting. Multiple genes from numerous genetic loci interact with one another to determine genetic predisposition. Further the interplay between genetic predisposition and environmental modulation is an unpredictable vital step in determining disease causation. All these are still ill understood from a purely scientific viewpoint though the rate of scientific progress is astonishing. Evidence suggests that **family history contributes to an increased risk of CVD** independently of the known environmental risk factors. Highrisk families make up a considerable proportion of early CVD cases in the general population. In one study, families with a history of early CVD represented only 14% of the general population but accounted for 72% of early CVD cases (men aged <55 years, women aged <65 years) and 48% of CVD at all ages. **A history of early CVD in a firstdegree relative approximately doubles the risk of CVD.** The promise of genetic studies is that it allows us: **(1)** To identify individuals at birth whose lifetime environmental risk exposure could be modulated genetically to mitigate CVD risk (the political and ethical ramifications of which are enormous) **(2)** To identify genetic disease mechanisms hitherto unknown that cause CHD and mitigate or block these pathways using disease specific drugs and/or environmental or behavioral change. In terms of human studies, traditional risk factors such as age, sex, smoking, and a family history of premature coronary heart disease are still more predictive of CAD than human genetic markers and genetic scores. Aging affects all metabolic processes and has a profound effect on atherosclerosis, and we do not yet fully understand the impact of aging at the cellular level. Thus, a clinical history is still especially useful. Let us therefore take heart and encourage everyone to: **(A)** Not lose hope but embrace knowledge and strive to understand their own cardiovascular risk level. We enclose with this book **a series of online sites and cellular phone apps** that easily and quickly enable one to **calculate their cardiovascular risk** – we encourage our readers to use them. **(B)** Act practically on the information provided by reducing their preventable risks– stop smoking, eat sensibly, increase physical activity, control lipids, regulate high blood pressure and manage diabetes...

**(C)** Help others by educating your family and friends: start with your children at home and at school but setting the right example – so much of what adults think is their favorite or desired life – style is influenced by familial and societal experience as a child at home and at school. The copious amounts of soda and pizza consumed by American school children every day is testament to my point. (D) We need better role models in advertising–less of the Marlboro man and more of the Marathon man. The irony is that America has exported not only Coke and Blue Jeans to the world, but the hamburger which is the iconic symbol of a cardiovascular time bomb. While science scrambles to regulate this disease, humanity must catch up with and control this CVD epidemic. To do this, we must first change attitudes then lifestyles. Let us start with awareness and export education and understanding before goods to developing countries, so that they do not have to relive the mistakes made in Western Europe and America over the last century. Those that neglect this aspect of medical history are condemned repeatedly to relieve its disastrous consequences.

Patients frequently ask: Many of us lead **an irregular lifestyle: working late, not enough we sleep, drink too much alcohol. Can it affect our heart?**

Lack of sleep, emotional stress, late hours, poor sleep and excess alcohol all translate into a poor CVD risk profile and hence adverse outcomes. The effects of alcohol are complex and biphasic, that is some may indeed be beneficial, but more is not necessarily better. Hence the cynical medical joke, "Don't drink more than your doctor spills". Drinking a glass of wine is good for the heart in the sense that it is believed alcohol protects the heart by increasing cardioprotective HDL or highdensity lipoprotein cholesterol. The grape skin provides flavonoids and other antioxidant substances that protect the heart and vessels from the damaging effects of oxygen free radicals (damaging inflammatory by products of metabolism) produced by our body and is antithrombotic. A glass of wine can reduce stress by promoting relaxation and pleasure. The strongest beneficial evidence is in favor of wine, but some evidence has also shown that beer and other types of alcohol may provide similar benefit. Like all good things, there is also a danger in excess use. **Alcohol in moderation does not seem to have an adverse effect, unless a persistently excessive amount is used, when the risks of high blood pressure, stroke, obesity, and cirrhosis of the liver supervene.** For all people, alcohol can lower blood sugar. So, for people with diabetes, it is recommended that any alcohol be consumed with a meal. In all cases, alcohol still contains calories, so remember to include it in the meal plan (one alcoholic drink is 1 fat exchange unit). **Drinking too much alcohol can raise the levels of some fats in the blood (triglycerides).** It can also lead to high blood pressure, heart failure and increased calorie intake. Consuming too many calories can lead to obesity and a higher risk of developing diabetes. Excessive drinking and binge drinking can also lead to stroke. Other serious problems include fetal alcohol syndrome when used in pregnancy, alcoholic cardiomyopathy, cardiac arrhythmia, cirrhosis, liver failure, and sudden cardiac death.

**Is there a link between heart disease and blood sugar?**

Diabetes is a disease that leads to high levels of blood sugar (glucose). It happens when the body does not make any or enough insulin or does not use insulin well. The link between diabetes (impaired blood sugar control) is one of the most challenging and important problems confronting the health of developing and developed countries.

A recent study (NHANES) in the Journal of American Medical Association (JAMA) examined the prevalence of diabetes and prediabetes and related disease trends in **U.S. adults from 19882012.**

**Prediabetes, also called impaired glucose tolerance (IGT) or impaired fasting glucose (IFG), is a condition in which your blood glucose levels are higher than normal but not high enough for a diagnosis of diabetes.** Having prediabetes puts you at higher risk of developing type 2 diabetes, heart disease and stroke. In addition to IGT and IFG, other factors that make it more likely a person will develop type 2 diabetes include:

- **Family history of diabetes** (i.e., parent, brother, or sister)
- **Ethnic/racial groups** like African Americans, Hispanic/Latinos, Asian Americans, Pacific Islanders, American Indians, and Alaska Natives
- Being morbidly overweight or obese (especially BMI>35)
- **Age 45 or older**
- **Women with a prior history of gestational diabetes** (diabetes diagnosed during pregnancy) or a baby weighing 9 pounds or more at birth
- **High blood pressure** or taking medicine for high blood pressure (especially thiazide diuretics)
- **Abnormal cholesterol (lipid) levels**
- **Inadequate physical activity**
- **Polycystic ovary syndrome (PCOS)**
- **Blood vessel problems** affecting the heart, brain or legs (cardiovascular disease)
- Presence of dark, thick, and velvety patches of skin
- around your neck or armpits (**acanthosis nigricans**)

One of the most startling findings in the **NHANES study** was that **more than half of American adults aged 20 or older in 2012 had either diabetes (14.3 percent of total population) or prediabetes (38.0 percent).** More than one-ethird of those who met the study's criteria for diabetes were completely unaware they had the disease. One of the most startling findings was that using the hemoglobin A1c, FPG or 2hour PG definition, more than half of Americans age 20 or older in 2012 had either diabetes (14.3 percent of total population) or prediabetes (38.0 percent). **More than 36 percent of those who met the study's criteria for diabetes, or an estimated 5 percent of the overall population, were unaware they had diabetes.** Researchers found diabetes was more prevalent among Hispanics (22.6 percent of all Hispanic participants), blacks (21.8 percent) and Asians (20.6 percent) compared with whites (11.3 percent). Asian Americans also had the highest percentage of undiagnosed cases (50.9 percent of total diabetes cases in this group).

Overall, the study found that diabetes rates increased from 9.8 percent of the total U.S. population in 198894 to 12.4 percent in 201112 across all age and racial/ethnic groups, in both genders, and by all education and income levels. **The incidence of new onset Diabetes and Obesity continue to rise in parallel.**

### Why has this epidemic occurred?

Our reliance on saturated fat, refined sugars, fructose laden drinks and sedentary lifestyle has pushed us in the direction of metabolic disaster. If I said one of three children born will develop a potentially fatal condition (e.g. HIV disease) during their lifetime, or that one in four adults over the age of 65 years will contract this disease every adult would be outraged and petition with their government representatives to stop it, and rightly so–yet this creeping epidemic has overwhelmed us, and many are unaware of it! **The best news is that we can do something about it and better still prevent it.** One of the most telling pieces of evidence for this statement comes from the **Diabetes Prevention Program (DPP), a major clinical trial aimed at discovering whether either diet and exercise or the oral diabetes drug metformin could prevent or delay the onset of type 2 diabetes in people with impaired glucose tolerance (IGT).** The results of the Diabetes Prevention Program showed that people with prediabetes who lose weight and increase their physical activity can prevent or delay type 2 diabetes. **The DPP's striking results tell us that millions of highrisk people can modify their diet and exercise to lose a small amount of weight to delay or prevent the development of type 2 diabetes. The DPP also suggests that metformin and more recently drugs called SGLT2 inhibitors, GLP1 agonists can be effective in delaying the onset of diabetes in predisposed people.** Participants in the lifestyle intervention group– those receiving intensive counseling on effective diet, exercise, and behavior modification–reduced their risk of developing diabetes by 58 percent. This finding was true across all participating ethnic groups and for both men and women. **Lifestyle changes** worked particularly well for participants aged 60 and older, reducing their risk by 71 percent. About 5 percent of the lifestyle intervention group developed diabetes each year during the study period, compared with 11 percent in those who did not get the intervention. Researchers believe that weight loss **achieved through better eating habits and exercise reduces the risk of diabetes by improving the ability of the body to use insulin and process glucose. Participants taking metformin reduced their risk of developing diabetes by 31 percent.** Metformin was effective for both men and women, but it was least effective in people aged 45 and older. Metformin was most effective in people 25 to 44 years old and in those with a body mass index of 35 or higher (at least 60 pounds overweight). About 7.8 percent of the metformin group developed diabetes each year during the study, compared with 11 percent of the group receiving the placebo. **Metformin (and potentially SGLT2 inhibitors) used in conjunction with strict diet and weight loss early in prediabetes or type 2 diabetes can retard the progression of diabetes** (preventing the onset of full diabetes in up to a third of people) and **prevent organ damage** including kidney failure, damaging heart wall thickening (left ventricular hypertrophy) and prevent heart attacks and death. To summarize, the link between sugar, lipids, weight gain and heart disease is essential to our understanding of the metabolic threat facing our society and the epidemic of strokes, heart attacks, kidney failure, blindness, amputations, infections, and death that will inevitably follow.

## ASPIRIN AS A PREVENTATIVE THERAPY FOR CVD

The decision to use aspirin as a preventative therapy in cardiovascular disease was long promoted by physicians and endorsed by the lay public. Some 29 million people 40 and older were taking an aspirin a day despite having no known heart disease in 2017. About 6.6 million of them were doing so on their own — a doctor never recommended it. Nearly half of people over 70 who do not have heart disease — estimated at about 10 million — are taking daily aspirin for prevention. **Recently however new compelling data from three large clinical trials suggests that unless your risk of disease reaches a threshold level the RISKS outweigh the benefits.** Three large studies challenged the dogma of routine preventative aspirin therapy. These studies are some of the largest and longest to test aspirin in people at low and moderate risk of a heart attack, and found **only marginal benefit** if any, especially for older adults.

### In the Aspirin to Reduce Risk of Initial Vascular Events

**(ARRIVE)** trial, more than 12,000 European and U.S. adults 55 years or older without diabetes were randomized to take 100 mg of entericcoated aspirin or placebo daily for a median followup of five years. The researchers for the ARRIVE trial enrolled participants determined to be at a moderate risk of CVD (participants' mean atherosclerotic CVD risk score was 17.3% to 17.4%). No difference occurred was found in the out – come of cardiovascular death, myocardial infarction, unstable angina, stroke, or transient ischemic attack. However,

1% of the aspirin group experienced gastrointestinal bleeding com – pared with only 0.5% of the placebo group.

The **ASCEND (A Study of Cardiovascular Events In Diabetes)** trial enrolled 15,000 adults 40 years or older with diabetes in primary care practice. After a mean followup of 7.4 years, a lower percentage of the aspirin group experienced serious vascular events than the placebo group, but this benefit was offset by an increased percentage of major bleeding events.

The number needed to treat was 91 to prevent a single vascular event and number needed to harm was 112 to cause a major bleeding event, from which it can be concluded that aspirin provided no net benefit.

Finally, the **ASPirin in Reducing Events in the Elderly (ASPREE)** trial examined the effect of five years of daily low-dose aspirin therapy on 19,114 relatively healthy community – dwelling adults 70 years or older in the United States and Australia. There were no differences in the primary endpoint of disabilityfree survival (death, dementia, and persistent physical disability) or cardiovascular deaths/ events, and hospitalizations. However, **the aspirin group had a significantly higher rate of major hemorrhage and higher mortality.**

**For these reasons, people over 70 who do not have heart disease — or are younger but at increased risk of bleeding should avoid daily aspirin for prevention.** The United States Preventative Services Task Force (USPSTF) recommends considering the initiation of lowdose aspirin use for primary prevention of cardiovascular disease (CVD) [and colorectal cancer] **only in adults aged 50 to 59 years who have a 10% or greater 10year CVD risk, are not at**

**increased risk for bleeding**, have a life expectancy of at least 10 years, and are willing to take lowdose aspirin daily for at least 10 years.

## CONGESTIVE HEART FAILURE

### What is congestive heart failure?

**Congestive heart failure (CHF) is a chronic progressive condition that affects the pumping power of the heart muscles.** While often referred to simply as "heart failure," CHF specifically refers to the disease in which fluid builds up in the lungs and extremities because the heart pumps inefficiently or poorly.

There are four heart chambers. The upper half of your heart has two atria, and the lower half of your heart has two ventricles. The ventricles pump blood to your body's organs and tissues, and the atria receive blood from the body as it circulates back from the organs and extremities. CHF develops when your ventricles organs and extremities can't pump blood in sufficient volume to the body. Eventually, blood and other fluids can back up collecting within several organs:

- **lungs**
- **abdomen**
- **liver**
- **lower extremities**

CHF can be lifethreatening. If you suspect you or some – one near you has CHF, seek immediate medical treatment.

## TYPES

### What are the most common types of CHF?

Leftsided CHF is the most common type of CHF. It occurs when the left ventricle doesn't efficiently or effectively pump blood around the body. As the condition progresses, fluid can build up in the lungs, which makes breathing difficult.

### There are two kinds of leftsided heart failure:

**Systolic heart failure** which occurs when the left ventricle fails to contract normally. This reduces the level of force available to pump blood into the circulation. Without this force, the heart can't pump effectively.

**Diastolic heart failure**, or diastolic dysfunction, happens when the muscle in the left ventricle becomes stiff. Because it can no longer relax properly, the heart cannot fill efficiently with blood between beats. The pressures inside the heart rise and fluid accumulation and overload results.

**Rightsided CHF** occurs when the right ventricle has dif ficulty pumping blood to your lungs. Blood backs up in your lower extremities and abdominal cavity causing abdominal swelling from internal fluid (called "ascites") and leg swelling called "edema".

A Holistic Approach to Understanding...

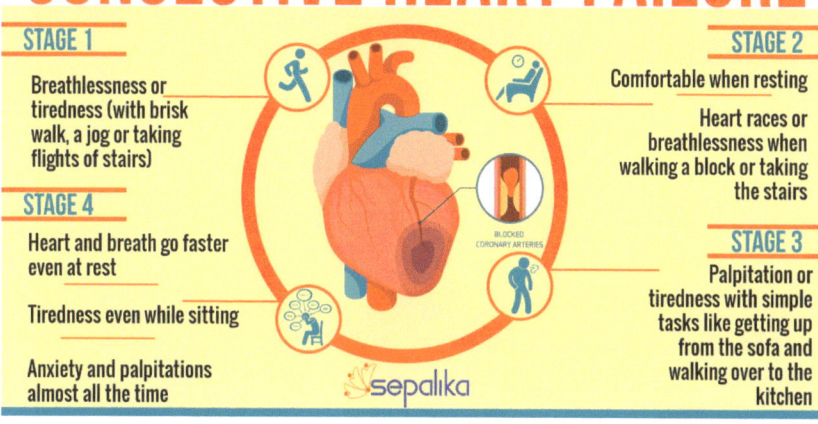

# THE FOUR STAGES OF CONGESTIVE HEART FAILURE

**STAGE 1**
Breathlessness or tiredness (with brisk walk, a jog or taking flights of stairs)

**STAGE 2**
Comfortable when resting

Heart races or breathlessness when walking a block or taking the stairs

**STAGE 3**
Palpitation or tiredness with simple tasks like getting up from the sofa and walking over to the kitchen

**STAGE 4**
Heart and breath go faster even at rest

Tiredness even while sitting

Anxiety and palpitations almost all the time

sepalika

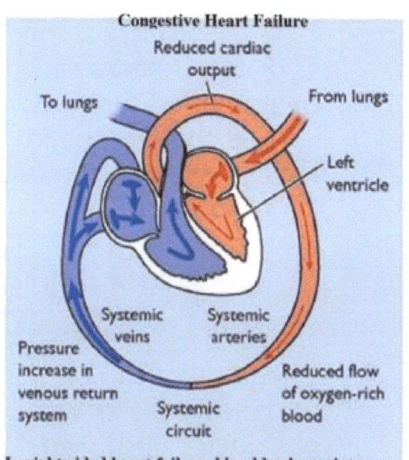

**Congestive Heart Failure**
- Reduced cardiac output
- To lungs
- From lungs
- Left ventricle
- Systemic veins
- Systemic arteries
- Pressure increase in venous return system
- Reduced flow of oxygen-rich blood
- Systemic circuit

In right-sided heart failure, blood backs up into systemic circulation, with JVD and pedal edema present.
Blood backs up into the lungs in left-sided heart failure, presenting with difficulty breathing and rales/crackles (fluid) lung sounds.

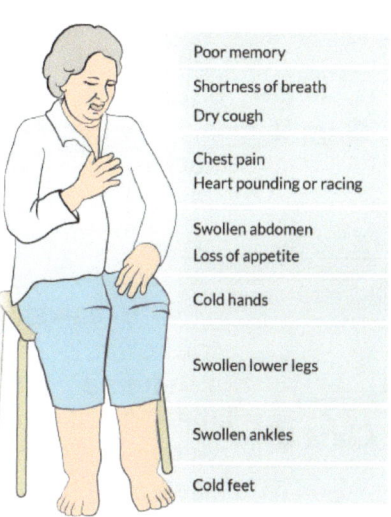

Poor memory

Shortness of breath

Dry cough

Chest pain

Heart pounding or racing

Swollen abdomen

Loss of appetite

Cold hands

Swollen lower legs

Swollen ankles

Cold feet

This results in fluid retention in your lower extremities, abdomen, and other vital organs.

It is possible to have leftsided and rightsided CHF at the same time. Usually, the disease starts on the left side and then involves the right when left untreated.

## Congestive heart failure stages

| Stage | Main symptoms | Outlook |
|---|---|---|
| Class I | You don't experience any symptoms during typical physical activity. | CHF at this stage can be managed through lifestyle changes, heart medications, and monitoring. |
| Class II | You're likely comfortable at rest, but normal physical activity may cause fatigue, palpitations, and shortness of breath. | CHF at this stage can be managed through lifestyle changes, heart medications, and careful monitoring. |
| Class III | You're likely comfortable at rest, but there's a noticeable limitation of physical activity. Even mild exercise may cause fatigue, palpitations, or shortness of breath. | Treatment can be complicated. Talk with your doctor about what heart failure at this stage may mean for you. |

| | | |
|---|---|---|
| **Class IV** | You're likely unable to carry on any amount of physical activity without symptoms, which are present even at rest. | There's no cure for CHF at this stage, but there are still quality-of-life and palliative care options. You'll want to discuss the potential benefits and risks of each with your doctor. |

## CHF CAUSES AND RISKS

### What are the causes of CHF, and am I at risk?

CHF may result from other health conditions that directly affect your cardiovascular system. This is why it's important to get annual checkups to lower your risk for heart health problems, including high blood pressure (hypertension), coronary artery disease, and heart valve conditions.

### Hypertension

When your blood pressure is higher than normal over a prolonged period (**Hypertension**), it may lead to CHF. Hypertension has many different causes. Among them is the narrowing and hardening of your arteries ("**Atherosclerosis**"), which makes it harder for your blood to flow through them.

## Coronary artery disease

Cholesterol and other types of fatty substances can block the coronary arteries, which are the small arteries that supply blood to the heart muscle. This causes the arteries to become narrow. Narrower coronary arteries restrict the blood flow to your organs and can lead to damage.

## Cardiac Valve conditions

Your heart valves regulate blood flow through your heart by opening and closing to let blood in and out of the chambers in a specific direction. Valves that don't open and close correctly may force your ventricles to work harder to pump blood. This can be a result of a heart infection, inflammatory damage, autoimmune diseases, or birth defects. **Any valve malfunction can deteriorate over time to heart failure and requires careful monitoring over time.**

## Other conditions

While heartrelated diseases can lead to CHF, there are other seemingly unrelated conditions that may increase your risk, too. These include diabetes, thyroid disease, and obesity. Severe infections and allergic reactions may also result in acute or chronic CHF.

In the early stages of CHF, the patient most likely notices little or subtle changes in health quality and symptoms. As the condition worsens, gradual changes in body function multiply with progressive deterioration occurring if uncorrected. Look for the cardinal **CHF symptoms and signs: Fatigue** (excessive and unusual), **swelling** of the ankles and feet, weight gain that is water not fat, shortness of breath with increasingly less exercise tolerance. Seek medical attention and do not put it off till a crisis supervenes!

## What are the symptoms of CHF?

| Symptoms you may notice first | Symptoms that indicate your condition has worsened | Symptoms that indicate a severe heart condition |
|---|---|---|
| fatigue | irregular heartbeat | chest pain that radiates through the upper body |
| swelling in your ankles, feet, and legs | a cough that develops from congested lungs | rapid breathing |
| weight gain | wheezing | skin that appears blue, which is due to lack of oxygen in your lungs |
| increased need to urinate, especially at night | shortness of breath, which may indicate pulmonary edema | fainting |

**Chest pain** that radiates through the upper body can also be a sign of a narrowed or blocked coronary artery or even a myocardial infarction or heart attack. If you experience this or any of the other symptoms that persist or worsen that may suggest point to a severe heart condition, **seek immediate medical attention.**

## DIAGNOSIS

### How is CHF diagnosed?

After reporting cardiac symptoms to a doctor, you may be referred to a heart/vascular specialist, known as a cardiologist. The cardiologist will perform a physical exam. The exam may involve listening to your heart with a stethoscope or obtaining an ECG to detect abnormal heart rhythms. To confirm an initial diagnosis, your cardiologist might also order certain diagnostic tests such as an echocardiogram (cardiac ultrasound) to examine your heart's valves, blood vessels, and chambers.

Tests your cardiologist may recommend:

An **electrocardiogram** (EKG or ECG) records your heart's rhythm. Abnormalities in your heart's rhythm, such as a rapid heartbeat or irregular rhythm, and thickening of the walls of the cardiac chambers can be suggested by an ECG. That could be a warning sign for a heart attack. ECG's can yield valuable signs of heart muscle ischemia (lack of nutritive blood flow), prior heart muscle injury, and acts as a timely warning for further investigation and corrective action.

An **echocardiogram** uses sound waves to record the heart's structure and motion. The test can determine if you already have poor blood flow, muscle damage, malfunctioning heart valves, abnormalities of the pericardium (the sac in which the heart sits), or a poorly functioning or stiff thickened myocardium (heart muscle that doesn't contract normally.

An **MRI scanner** takes pictures of your heart. With both still and moving pictures, and no ionizing radiation, this allows a convenient highresolution imaging technique to see if there is damage to the heart muscle, valve or pericardial malfunction or abnormal deficient coronary artery blood flow.

**MRI imaging** is destined to replace many forms of cardiac testing that involve recurrent exposure to ionizing radioactive isotopes conventionally used for nuclear stress tests.

**Stress tests** show how well your heart performs under different levels of physiological stress. Making your heart work harder under conditions of exercise, makes it easier for your doctor to diagnose problems that occur in real life. **Stress tests can involve nuclear isotope imaging that allows pictures of the heart muscle blood flow to be captured by a gamma scanner technology, and compared while monitoring the ECG during, before and after exercise** (or after intravenous infusion of medicine that dilates the coronary arteries). The differences in imaged blood flow are interpreted for probability of coronary artery flow limitation or coronary atherosclerotic blockages.

Blood tests can check for abnormal blood cells and infections. Blood tests can also check the level of BNP, a hormone that rises with heart failure.

**Cardiac catheterization** can directly demonstrate blockages of the coronary arteries. The physician will insert a small tube called a "catheter" into a blood vessel (artery or vein) and thread it from your upper thigh (groin area), arm, or wrist to the heart over a guidewire. At this time, the doctor can take blood samples, use Xrays to view your coronary arteries, and check coronary artery blood flow and obstructions, as well as check blood pressure in your heart chambers and heart muscle function. All this data is then used to determine the overall flow status in the coronary arteries, the flow function of the heart valves, and the contractile status of the heart muscle. It is however an invasive study albeit with low risk in noncritically ill patients. Nevertheless, noninvasive screening tests are usually employed prior to cardiac catheterization to avoid unnecessary invasive procedures.

## TREATMENT

| Symptom | Action |
|---|---|
| Best weight: _____ <br> If you have: <br> • No trouble breathing <br> • No chest pain <br> • No weight change overnight or over the last week <br> • The usual amount of ankle swelling <br> • No change in ability to be active | Your symptoms are under control. <br> • Keep taking your medications every day, as ordered <br> • Keep weighing yourself every day and writing down your weight <br> • Follow a low-salt diet <br> • Keep all your medical appointments |
| If you: <br> • Need more pillows than usual to sleep <br> • Have more trouble breathing when you are active <br> • Have more coughing than usual <br> • Increased shortness of breath with activity <br> • Gain 2 to 3 pounds overnight, or 5 pounds in one week <br> • Have more swelling than usual | You might need to take extra medicine. <br><br> Call your doctor's office to find out what you should do. <br><br> Doctor name: _____ <br> Phone #: _____ |
| If you: <br> • Have trouble breathing when you are resting, or you can't stop coughing <br> • Wheeze or feel chest tightness when you are resting <br> • Wake up at night because you can't breathe well <br> • Feel dizzy, very tired, or like you might fall <br> • Gain or lose more than 5 pounds compared to your normal weight | You probably need to **see** a doctor right away. <br><br> Call your doctor **now**. <br><br> Doctor name: _____ <br> Phone #: _____ |

A Holistic Approach to Understanding…

If you:
- Have trouble breathing that does not get better no matter what you do
- Feel like you can't breathe, or start to turn blue
- Cough up frothy or pink saliva
- Have pain or pressure in your chest, or you have other signs of a heart attack
- Have a fast or uneven heartbeat that will not go away or makes you feel dizzy or lightheaded
- Feel very confused
- Faint

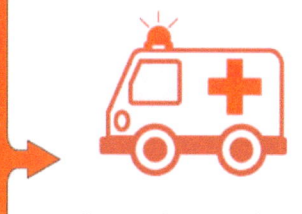

Call 9-1-1 for an ambulance **right away**

## ZONES TO MANAGE HEART FAILURE

| | You have: | What to do: |
|---|---|---|
|  **GREEN ZONE** | ♥ No shortness of breath<br>♥ No weight gain more than 3 pounds per day<br>♥ No swelling of feet, ankles, legs or stomach<br>♥ No chest pain | ♥ Keep up the good work!<br>♥ Take your medicine<br>♥ Eat a low salt diet<br>♥ Weigh yourself every day |
| 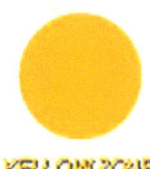 **YELLOW ZONE** | ♥ Weight gain of 3 pounds in 1 day or 5 pounds in one week<br>♥ More shortness of breath<br>♥ More swelling in your feet, ankles, legs, or stomach<br>♥ Feeling more tired<br>♥ New or unusual coughing<br>♥ Dizziness<br>♥ Hard to breathe lying down — need to sleep sitting in chair | ♥ Call your doctor or nurse |
| 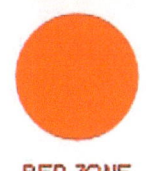 **RED ZONE** | ♥ Hard time breathing<br>♥ Struggling to breathe even at rest<br>♥ Chest pain or discomfort<br>♥ Feeling faint | ♥ Call 911 or<br>♥ Get help, go to Emergency Room |

# HEART FAILURE ZONES

## EVERY DAY

- Weigh yourself in the morning before breakfast. Write it down. Compare your weight today to your weight yesterday.
- Keep the total amount of fluids you drink to only 6 to 8 glasses each day. (6-8 glasses equals 1500-2000 mL or 48-64 oz)
- Take your medicine exactly how your doctor said.
- Check for swelling in your feet, ankles, legs, and stomach.
- Eat foods that are low in salt or salt-free.
- Balance activity and rest periods.

## WHICH ZONE ARE YOU IN TODAY?

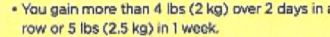

### GREEN SAFE ZONE

**ALL CLEAR – This zone is your goal!**

Your symptoms are under control. You have:
- No shortness of breath.
- No chest discomfort, pressure, or pain.
- No swelling or increase in swelling of your feet, ankles, legs, or stomach.
- No weight gain of more than 4 lbs (2 kg) over 2 days in a row or 5 lbs (2.5 kg) in 1 week.

### YELLOW CAUTION ZONE

**CAUTION – This zone is a warning**

Call your Health Care provider (eg. Doctor, nurse) if you have any of the following:
- You gain more than 4 lbs (2 kg) over 2 days in a row or 5 lbs (2.5 kg) in 1 week.
- You have vomiting and/or diarrhea that lasts more than two days.
- You feel more short of breath than usual.
- You have increased swelling in your feet, ankles, legs, or stomach.
- You have a dry hacking cough.
- You feel more tired and don't have the energy to do daily activities.
- You feel lightheaded or dizzy, and this is new for you.
- You feel uneasy, like something does not feel right.
- You find it harder for you to breathe when you are lying down.
- You find it easier to sleep by adding pillows or sitting up in a chair.

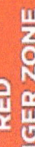
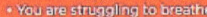

### RED DANGER ZONE

**EMERGENCY – This zone means act fast!**

Go to emergency room or call 9-1-1 if you have any of the following:
- You are struggling to breathe.
- Your shortness of breath does not go away while sitting still.
- You have a fast heartbeat that does not slow down when you rest.
- You have chest pain that does not go away with rest or with medicine.
- You are having trouble thinking clearly or are feeling confused.
- You have fainted.

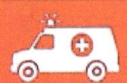

## Treatments

- Blood Pressure Medications: to decrease workload of the heart.
- Diuretics: Medications to help control fluid build up in the body.
- Coronary Bypass Surgery
- Valve Replacement or Repair
- Lifestyle changes:
    - Daily Weights (to monitor fluid retention
    - Smoking Cessation
    - Salt Restriction in the diet
    - Limit high fat foods and alcohol

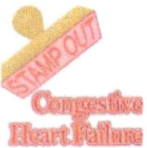

### How is heart failure treated?

You and your doctor may consider different treatments depending on your overall health and how far your condition has progressed.

### Congestive heart failure drugs

There are several medications that can be used to treat CHF, including:

Angiotensinconverting enzyme inhibitors (ACE inhibitors) open up narrowed blood vessels to improve blood flow. Other vasodilators (medicines that dilate the blood vessels) are another option if you cannot tolerate ACE inhibitors.

**ACE inhibitors** have been shown to be effective in treating blood pressure as well as improving survival and quality of life in CHF patients. They can protect the kidneys from damage from blood pressure (hypertension) and diabetes.

**They are important medications therapeutically.**

The following **ACE inhibitors** are used commonly in the United States and Europe:
- benazepril
- captopril
- enalapril
- fosinopril
- lisinopril
- quinapril
- ramipril
- moexipril
- perindopril
- trandolapril

ACE inhibitors should be taken with the following medications only after careful consideration with a doctor, as they may cause an adverse reaction:

Thiazide diuretics can cause an additional decrease in blood pressure and are often synergistically combined with ACE inhibitors. Potassiumsparing diuretics, such as triamterene, eplerenone, and spironolactone, are useful in combi – nation with thiazide diuretics but can cause potassium buildup in blood. **This may lead to abnormal heart rhythms if the potassium levels are excessively high.** It should be monitored for periodically using laboratory tests by your physician. **Nonsteroidal antiinflammatory drugs (NSAID)**, such as ibuprofen, aspirin, and naproxen, can cause sodium and water retention. This may reduce the ACE inhibitor's effect on your blood pressure. When NSAIDS are used routinely long term, they promote hypertension, deterioration of kidney function, exacerbate CHF, and **significantly increase the risk of stomach ulcers, and risk of myocardial infraction** (heart attack). Always be guided in long term NSAID use by your physician.

Betablockers can reduce blood pressure and slow a rapid heart rhythm.
- acebutolol
- atenolol
- bisoprolol
- carvedilol
- esmolol
- metoprolol
- nadolol
- nebivolol
- propranolol

Betablockers should be taken with caution with the following medications, as they may cause adverse reactions:
- Antiarrhythmic medications, such as amiodarone, can increase cardiovascular effects, including reduced blood pressure and slow heart rate (bradycardia).
- Antihypertensive medications, such as lisinopril (Zestril), losartan, and aldactone, may also increase the likelihood of cardiovascular sideeffects, when used together
- The effects of albuterol on bronchodilation may be cancelled out by betablockers. **Betablockers can precipitate asthmatic crises in brittle asthmatics and should be avoided in brittle asthmatics.**

- Antipsychotics, such as thioridazine, may also cause low blood pressure, as may many psychoactive antianxiety, antidepression medications
- Clonidine may cause low blood pressure, drowsiness, fatigue, dry eyes/mouth, irritability, insomnia, nightmares and constipation
- **Diuretics** reduce your body's fluid content. CHF can cause your body to retain more fluid than it should. Diuretics generally cause the loss of sodium and water in the urine and in some case have relaxing properties on the blood vessels even in low dose.

Your doctor may recommend many CHF medications including:

- **Thiazide diuretics.** These cause blood vessels to relax and help the body remove any extra fluid. Examples include metolazone, chlorthalidone, indapamide, and hydrochlorothiazide. These can be used alone or in conjunction with loop diuretics.
- **Loop diuretics.** These are strong diuretics and cause the
- kidneys to produce more urine. This helps remove excess fluid from your body. Examples include furosemide, ethacrynic acid, bumetanide,
- Potassiumsparing diuretics. This helps get rid of fluids and sodium while still retaining potassium. Examples include triamterene, eplerenone, and spironolactone.
- **Diuretics** should be taken with caution with the following medications, as they may interact and cause an adverse reaction:

- **ACE inhibitors**, such as lisinopril (Zestril), benazepril, and captopril, can cause cough, decreased blood pressure, elevated potassium levels, and even kidney failure especially if the patient is dehydrated.
- **Tricyclic antidepressants**, such as amitriptyline and desipramine, may cause low blood pressure, drowsiness, dry mouth, blurred vision, constipation, mental confusion.
- **Anxiolytics**, such as alprazolam, chlordiazepoxide, and diazepam, may cause low blood pressure, dizziness and drowsiness.
- **Hypnotics,** such as zolpidem and triazolam, may cause low blood pressure and respiratory depression if used in large doses or with other sedatives or alcohol which can be fatal.
- **Betablockers,** such as acebutolol and atenolol, may cause low blood pressure, fatigue, and erectile dysfunction.
- **Calcium channel** blockers, such as amlodipine and diltiazem, may cause a drop in blood pressure and ankle swelling or edema.
- Nitrates, such as nitroglycerin and isosorbidedinitrate, may cause low blood pressure and headache.
- **NSAIDS**, such as ibuprofen, aspirin, and naproxen, may cause water retention, high blood pressure, liver and kidney toxicity.

## Surgeries

If medications aren't effective on their own, more invasive procedures may be required. Angioplasty, a procedure to open blocked arteries, is one option. The cardiologist may also consider **heart valve repair surgery to restore normal valve function** and improve cardiac function. Many heart valve surgeries are now accomplished using percutaneous **minimally invasive catheter techniques** to either open (stent open) narrowed valves or clip and restore function of leaking valves.

### What can I expect in the long term?

Your condition may improve with medication or surgery. The outlook depends on how advanced the CHF is and whether there are other health conditions to treat, such as diabetes or hypertension. **The earlier the CHF condition is diagnosed, the better the outlook will be.** Your physician will determine the best treatment plan individualized to your needs. Beneficial treatment pathways are usually avail – able with current medical progress.

## CHF PREVENTION
### How to prevent congestive heart failure

There are several things you can do to lower your risk of heart failure, or at least delay CHF onset. You can:
- **Avoid or quit smoking**. If you do smoke and have not been able to quit, ask your doctor to recommend

products and services that can help. **Secondhand smoke is also a health hazard.** If you live with a smoker, help them to quit and always ask them to smoke outdoors. **Ecigarettes and vaping inhalation should be AVOIDED at all costs.**
- **Maintain a wellbalanced diet.** A hearthealthy diet is rich in vegetables, fruits, and whole grains. Dairy products should be lowfat or fatfree. You also need protein in your diet. Things to avoid include salt (sodium), excess carbohydrates, added sugars, saturated and transfats, and refined grains.
- **Exercise.** As little as one hour of moderate aerobic exercise
- per week can improve your heart health. Walking, bicycling, and swimming are good forms of exercise. If you have not exercised in a while, start with just **15 minutes a day** and work your way up. If you feel unmotivated to work out alone, consider taking a class or signing up for personal training at a local gym. **Walking truly helps a CHF patient live longer.** Do something however small it may seem but do it regularly and build on your progress!
- **Watch your weight**. Being too heavy can be hard on your heart. Follow a balanced diet and exercise regularly. If you are not at a healthy weight, talk to your doctor and dietician about how to reduce weight with a safe weight loss program. Consulting with a dietician or nutritionist can be valuable. Excess weight increases CV risk globally through a variety of mechanisms

including elevated BP, elevated lipids, increased diabetic tendency, development of sleep apnea, and by promoting physical inactivity.
- **Be careful.** Drinking is to be regarded as a pleasurable
- habit that in moderation under specific circumstances, may have health benefits. It is not to be treated a universal panacea of health though it must be admitted it is pleasurable for the soul. **Drink alcohol (if you must) only in moderation and stay away from illegal drugs.** When taking prescription medications, follow instructions carefully and never increase your dose without doctor supervision.

If you are at high risk for heart failure or already have some heart damage, you can still follow these steps. Be sure to ask your doctor how much physical activity is safe and if you have any other restrictions. If you are on medication for high blood pressure, heart disease, or diabetes, take them exactly as directed. **Make sure to see your doctor regularly to monitor your condition and report any new symptoms right away to your physician.**

## ATRIAL FIBRILLATION

### WHAT IS ATRIAL FIBRILLATION?

The heart has four chambers, which usually beat in a steady rhythm. An abnormal heart rhythm, or arrhythmia, is when the heart does not beat in a steady or regular pattern. Atrial fibrillation (AF) is one common type of arrhythmia. AF occurs when the upper chambers of the heart (the atria) fibrillate, or "quiver," which causes a rapid, irregular heart rhythm. The normal heart rate for an adult is between 60 and 100 beats every minute. When the heart is in AF, the atria can beat over 300 times every minute. AF itself is not dangerous; however, **if left untreated, the side effects of AF can be lifethreatening.** When the atria are fibrillating, the flow of blood to the lower chambers of the heart (the ventricles) is slowed and stagnant, which increases the risk of a blood clot forming. **If a blood clot were to break loose, it could result in a stroke, a heart attack, or death**. Without treatment, AF can also cause the ventricles to beat too fast. Over time, this can weaken the heart muscle and lead to heart failure. AF is the most com – mon type of arrhythmia. There are approximately 2.3 million people in the United States who have AF, with 160,000 new cases diagnosed every year. Approximately nine out of every 100 people over the age of 65 have AF. Although it usually occurs in people older than 60, younger people can develop AF, too.

**The Cardiac Electrical System and Atrial Fibrillation**

The electrical system of the heart is the power source that makes the heartbeat. Electrical impulses travel along a pathway in the heart and make the atria and the ventricles work together to pump blood through the heart. A normal heartbeat begins with an electrical impulse in the sinoatrial (SA) node, a small bundle of tissue located in the right atrium. The impulse sends out an electrical pulse that causes both atria to contract (squeeze) and move blood into the ventricles.

The electrical current then passes through a small bundle of tissue called the atrioventricular (AV) node (the electrical bridge between the upper and lower chambers of the heart), which makes the ventricles squeeze (contract) and release in a steady rhythm. As the chambers relax and contract, they draw blood into the heart and push it back out to the rest of the body.

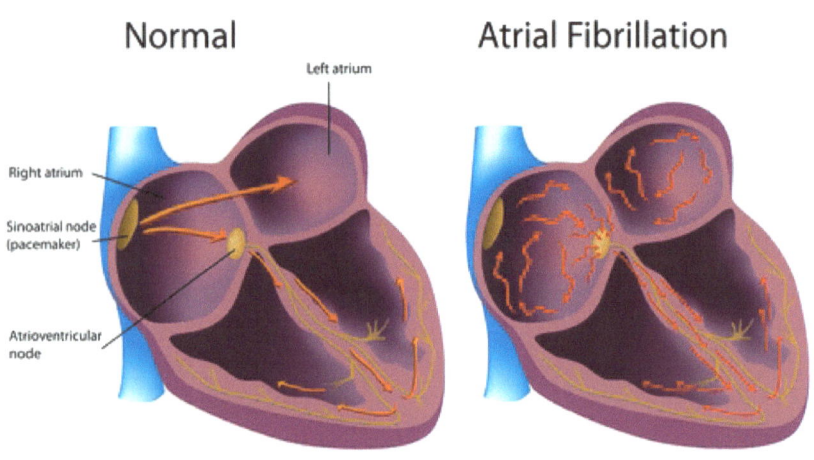

This is what causes the pulse we feel on our wrist or neck. **AF occurs when the atria begin to fibrillate, or "quiver," rapidly, and therefore do not contract effectively.** Instead of one electrical impulse moving through the heart, many impulses begin chaotically in the atria and fight to get through the AV node. There are several factors that allow this abnormal electrical rhythm to occur and continue. Certain medical conditions, such as poorly treated high blood pressure (hypertension), coronary artery disease, and heart valve disease, can change the electrical proper – ties within the heart, making it more likely for AF to occur. Many of these conditions become more common as people age. **Many middle aged and older people have AF without knowing it.** As the electrical path way changes, one or more "triggers" may develop. Triggers are electrical circuits that send extra impulses at a fasterthanusual rate. These extra impulses induce the atria to fibrillate, or "quiver," in a fast and disorganized way.

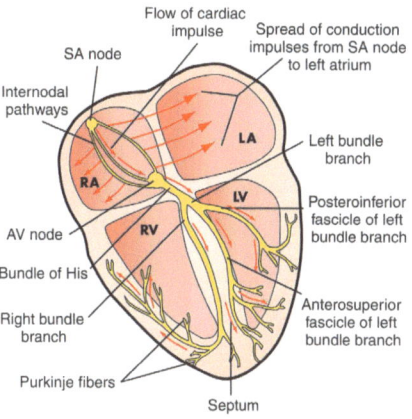

## Three Types of Atrial Fibrillation

**Paroxysmal AF** – Paroxysmal AF refers to AF that comes and goes on its own. The AF may last for seconds, minutes, hours, or even several days before the heart returns to its normal rhythm. People with this type of AF may have more symptoms than others. As the heart goes in and out of AF, the pulse rate may change from slow to fast and back again in short periods of time. **There is a definite risk of stroke in the presence of atrial fibrillation.**

**Persistent AF** – Persistent AF is when the AF does not stop by itself and lasts for more than 7 days. Medications or a special type of electrical shock (**cardioversion**) are needed to help the heart return to a normal rhythm. If no treatment is given, the heart will stay in AF. If the persistent AF lasts for more than 1 year, this type of AF is called longstanding persistent AF.

**Permanent AF** – Permanent AF is when a normal heart rhythm cannot be restored. Medications, procedures, and controlled electrical shocks do not help return the heart to a normal rhythm. In this condition there is an absolute need for anticoagulant for stroke prevention.

## Symptoms of Atrial Fibrillation

The symptoms of AF are different for each person. Some people with AF can tell as soon as AF begins. Others don't appear to have any troubling symptoms. They do not even know they have AF. This is because the symptoms depend on the rate of the heartbeat while in AF, the cause of AF (other heart problems, diseases, etc.), and on how much AF affects the pumping efficiency of the heart.

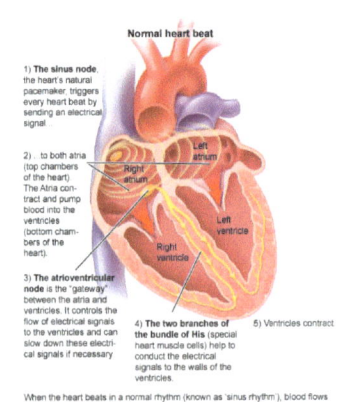

### The symptoms of AF:
- Feeling fatigued, excessively tired or not having enough energy (most common) for day to day tasks

- Having a pulse that is faster than normal or one that changes between fast and slow (**tachycardia-bradycardia** syndrome)
- Shortness of breath
- **Heart palpitations** (feeling like your heart is racing, pounding, or fluttering)
- **Unusual fatigue** and trouble with everyday exercises or activities
- **Chest pain**, chest pressure, tightness, or discomfort.
- **Dizziness or feeling lightheaded**
- **Fainting**
- **Increased urination.**

### How Is Atrial Fibrillation Diagnosed?

There are several tests that are done when someone has a fast or irregular heartbeat. Your doctor may order these tests if you are having signs or symptoms of a heart problem. The symptoms include heart palpitations (feeling like your heart is racing, pounding, or fluttering), shortness of breath, or dizziness. After a physical examination, your doctor may order one or more of the following tests:

**Electrocardiogram (ECG)** – An ECG is a snapshot of your heart's electrical activity. It is often performed in a doctor's office. Sticky conduction patches (electrodes) are attached to your chest, arms, and legs. These electrodes measure the rate and rhythm of your heart. An ECG is commonly used to diagnose AF. **Many smart wearable devices such as internet**

**and cellular connected watches (e.g. apple watch) now display a continuous real time ECG and allow the diagnosis of AF remotely by your physician.**

**Holter monitor** – **A Holter monitor is a portable continuous ECG.** It is typically worn for 24 hours but can be worn for several days. Stickers (electrodes) are placed on your chest and are then connected to a small recording machine that is usually worn around the waist. It records the electrical activity of your heart for 24 to 48 hours for your doctor to review later. A **continuous ECG monitor with patch ECG technology (event recorder**) that records information for 1030 days intermittently by patient activation is also available.

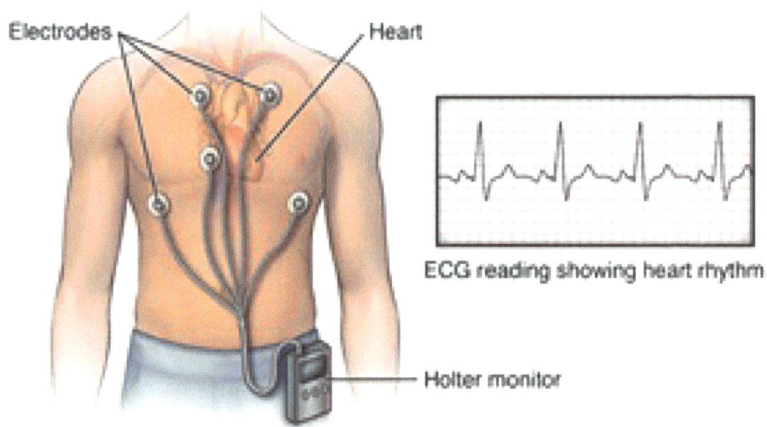

Holter monitor with ECG reading

**Mobile Cardiac Outpatient Telemetry (MCOT) – This is a continuous event monitor is like a Holter monitor but it is worn for up to 30 days**. It monitors your heartbeat when it is normal and will trigger a recording when it senses an abnormal rhythm (arrhythmia). The results are automatically sent to your doctor. Your physician will use this information to evaluate your symptoms and determine what is causing the arrhythmia. This type of monitor is helpful to diagnose AF in "asymptomatic" patients (people who do not have common symptoms) or in patients who have AF infrequently or only occasionally.

**Intermittent Event Monitor** – An intermittent event monitor is a portable ECG that is used for patients who have an irregular heart rhythm every occasionally. You will carry the monitor with you always and place it on your chest when you feel symptoms. This lets your doctor check your heart rhythm at the time of your symptoms. The recording can then be transmitted over the phone or internet for review.

**Implantable Loop Recorder – Implantable loop recorders (ILRs) are small devices that continuously record the heart's rate and rhythm.** The newer ILRs can be as small as a matchstick. These are implanted under the skin in the chest area. The ILR transmits information on your heart's rate and rhythm to a small standalone receiving unit that can be placed on a tabletop. Data are transmitted to a monitoring center that shares the information with your doctor. ILRs are mostly used for patients who have an irregular heart rhythm occasionally and unpredictably. The battery used in the ILR typically lasts three years.

Dr. Sanjay Srivatsa

## WEARABLE TECHNOLOGY IN THE DETECTION OF ATRIAL FIBRILLATION

Wearables are now a staple of modern life, with the global market set to double by 2022. **Mobile health (mHealth) devices** can be used for the diagnosis of atrial fibrillation. An estimated six million people in the United States, i.e. nearly 2 percent, have atrial fibrillation that results in an increased risk of events like clot (thrombus) embolization, heart attacks and strokes. It's thought that about 700,000 people with the condition don't know they have it. Early diagnosis allows better treatment and prevention of secondary diseases like stroke. Although there are many different mHealth devices to screen for atrial fibrillation, their accuracy varies due to differing technological approaches. Currently, either a sensor e.g. an optical sensor is used to monitor the pulse/circulation, or a direct skin contact method of ECG monitoring is used or a combination of both. In the largest study of this mHealth technology to date **Apple Heart Study**, 19,297 participants over 8 months underwent 117 days of monitoring, and 2161 participants (0.52%) received notifications of an irregular pulse. Among the 450 participants who returned analyzable ECG patches, **atrial fibrillation was present in 34% of participants 65 years of age or older**, or 153 people. Those 153 represented only 0.04 percent of the 420,000 participants. The ECGbased **AliveCor Kardia™ device** is an FDAapproved device. The AliveCor Kardia Mobile ECG is a singlechannel cardiac event recorder. It consists of a device and app that enables you to record and review electrocardiograms (ECG's) anywhere, anytime. The de – vice attaches to the back of most iOS and Android devices, and communicates wirelessly with its software application, providing display, analysis and communication capabilities. It has an extremely high overall accuracy and benefits from its ease of use. While the use of mHealth devices is convenient, after atrial fibrillation detection through an mHealth device, the diagnosis **should always be confirmed** by standard 12lead ECG, Holter monitoring and should lead to physician review and treatment considerations.

**Echocardiogram** – An echocardiogram uses sound waves to produce images of your heart. This test allows your doctor to see how the muscle, valves and chambers of your heart are working. There are two types of echocardiograms:

**Transthoracic echocardiogram (TTE)** – This is the standard echocardiogram that gives your doctor a picture of your beating heart. It is noninvasive, which means that there are no cuts, and nothing goes inside your body. A technician spreads a special transduction gel on your chest and then moves the ultrasound transducer, across your chest. The transducer picks up sound waves that reflect off the walls and valves in your heart. A computer then recreates a video image of your heart. This video can show the size of your heart, how well your heart is working, which walls are damaged, if the heart valves are working normally, and if there are blood masses or blood clots (thrombi) in your heart. **Transesophageal echocardiogram (TEE)** – A transesophageal echocardiogram, or **TEE**, is done when the doctor needs to get a good picture of the heart. A probe, called a transducer, is inserted through your mouth and moved down your esophagus (the tube that connects your mouth to your stomach). Having the transducer positioned in the esophagus allows for a clearer picture of the cardiac chambers due to lack of intervening body structures to obstruct the path of the ultrasound beam. The esophagus passes right behind the heart allowing a clear view of the heart unimpeded by the lungs and other tissues. This procedure can be uncomfortable, so a small amount of sedation through an intravenous (IV) line is given to make the patient less anxious and mildly drowsy. A topical spray is used to numb the back of your throat, so the transducer can be moved into the esophagus with minimal discomfort. Once the transducer is in place, it works the same way as described for transthoracic echocardiography. Since this test gives a better picture of the atria, **it is often used to rule out the presence of a blood clot in the heart in patients with AF, especially prior to cardioversion (electrical shock reversion of cardiac rhythm)**.

**Cardiac computerized tomography (CT)** – Cardiac computed tomography, or cardiac CT, uses an Xray machine and a computer to take fast automated, clear, detailed pictures of the heart in very thin sections. During a cardiac CT scan, you will lie on a table. An Xray machine will move around your body. The machine will take pictures of your heart and chest. A computer will put the pictures together to make a threedimensional (3D) picture of your heart and chest.

**Magnetic resonance imaging (MRI)** – A **Cardiac MRI** uses a powerful magnetic field generated by body enveloping magnets, and the generated radio wave signals from your body in response to the generated magnetic field to create a computer generated picture of your heart (or whatever body part is imaged). During a cardiac MRI, you will have to lie on a table inside a long tubelike machine for at least an hour (though taking breaks frequently in between). Cardiac MRI creates detailed pictures of your heart and can also take real time videos of your heart beating. Doctors use cardiac MRI to evaluate the beating heart, the chambers of the heart, the flow and pressures within the heart and can then determine in very detailed fashion, how well the heart is functioning.

**Risk Factors for Atrial Fibrillation**

Some people who have a healthy lifestyle and without any other medical problems develop AF. However, there are common causes and risk factors for AF:

- Age older than 60 years
- Heart problems
    - High blood pressure (hypertension)
    - Coronary artery disease
    - Prior heart attacks
    - Congestive heart failure
    - Structural heart disease (valve problems or congenital defects)
    - Previous openheart (valve or coronary bypass) surgery
    - **Untreated atrial flutter** (common abnormal heart rhythm that can deteriorate to AF and which needs anticoagulation)

- Diabetes
- Thyroid disease
- Chronic lung disease
- Sleep apnea
- Excessive alcohol or caffeine or stimulant use
- Recreational drug abuse
- Serious illness or infection
- Blood clots in the lung

**Complications from Atrial Fibrillation**

AF is usually not life threatening. However, **AF can have serious complications, including heart failure and stroke**. Thus, **AF needs to be treated whether you are having any symptoms or not.** To help prevent these complications, AF treatment includes medications to keep the pulse from going too fast and if possible, to keep the rhythm normal. In addition, **most patients need to take a medication (an anticoagulant) to prevent blood clots from forming in the heart** chambers and embolizing to the brain (stroke) or to the peripheral vital organs.

**Cardiomyopathy**

AF can cause a fast pulse rate for long periods of time. This causes the ventricles to beat too fast. When the ventricles beat too fast for long periods of time, the heart muscle weakens and then the heart dilates in size to compensate. This condition is called cardiomyopathy. **Cardiomyopathy**

**can lead to heart failure and longterm disability**. Because of the potential for a weakened heart muscle, it is important to make sure that the rate of heart contraction while in AF is not too fast or too slow. This may require medications to slow heart rate or a pacemaker to compensate for a slow heartbeat.

**Stroke**

The most common risk for people with AF is having blood clots form in the heart. **One out of every 4 strokes in the USA is due to Atrial Fibrillation. People with AF have a stroke risk that is 5 times higher than people who do not have AF.** When the atria are fibrillating, the flow of blood to the ventricles is slowed. Since blood is not pumping effectively, blood in the atria may pool and clot. If the clot is pumped out of the heart, it could travel to the brain and lead to a stroke. A **stroke caused by AF is severe and disabling** due to its unpredictable catastrophic nature. In addition, strokes caused by AF have double the mortality rate of strokes not caused by AF. Because of this, **stroke prevention is a primary treatment goal** for AF.

**Measuring Stroke Risk:**
**The CHA2DS2VASc Risk Scoring Tool**
Your stroke risk depends on your age and whether you have other risk factors for stroke, such as heart disease, high blood pressure (hypertension), diabetes, or vascular disease, among others. The **CHA2DS2VASc stroke risk tool** helps doctors quickly measure your risk of stroke. Points

are assigned for each major stroke risk factor. By adding the points, your doctor can quickly determine your stroke risk. Higher total points mean a higher risk of stroke. This calculator is available online or as an application on a smartphone.

## Preventing Stroke

If you have an increased risk for a stroke, your doctor may ask you to take **anticoagulant** medicine. These medications are sometimes called "blood thinners" and make it harder for your blood to clot.

Anticoagulation medications include warfarin, dabigatran, apixaban, and rivaroxaban. If you

have a low risk of stroke or cannot take anticoagulants, your doctor may recommend aspirin to prevent clots from forming.

| | |
|---|---|
| **C**ongestive heart failure<br>Signs/symptoms of heart failure confirmed with objective evidence of cardiac dysfunction | +1 |
| **H**ypertension<br>Resting BP > 140/90 mmHg on at least 2 occasions or current antihypertensive pharmacologic treatment | +1 |
| **A**ge 75 years or older | +2 |
| **D**iabetes mellitus<br>Fasting glucose > 125 mg/dL or treatment with oral hypoglycemic agent and/or insulin | +1 |
| **S**troke, TIA, or TE<br>Includes any history of cerebral ischemia | +2 |
| **V**ascular disease<br>Prior MI, peripheral arterial disease, or aortic plaque | +1 |
| **A**ge 65 to 74 years | +1 |
| **S**ex **C**ategory (female)<br>Female gender confers higher risk | +1 |

Aspirin does not offer the stroke protection that blood thinners do. **Anticoagulants are exceptionally good at preventing stroke.** However, these blood thinning medications increase the risk of excess bleeding. **Your doctor must carefully weigh the risks and benefits of blood thinners for you.**

**Only your physician can decide if the risk of a stroke from AF is higher than the risk of major bleeding from**

**blood thinning medicine.** For many patients, the risk of bleeding is small compared to the risk of stroke. In other words, many people with AF should take an anticoagulant. Anticoagulants do not work the same way for every person. Many factors, including other medications that you take and your diet, can affect how well they will work for you. As with any medical treatment, there are risks and side effects. **All patients should discuss the benefits and risks of the different anticoagulation medications and any drugdrug interactions with their doctor.**

## Measuring Bleeding Risk

There are several bleeding risk scoring tools, which help doctors measure your bleeding risk. Like stroke risk scoring tools, each risk factor for bleeding is given specific points. By adding the points, your doctor can determine your bleeding risk. Higher total points mean a higher risk of bleeding.

**It is common for people with a high stroke risk to also have a high bleeding risk.** In this case, you should talk to your doc – tor about your preferences and priorities. For many patients with AF, avoiding a disabling stroke is their top priority. Bleeding risk calculators like HASBLED are available online or using mobile software applications.

## Stroke Symptoms and Response

If you or someone you know experiences any of the following **stroke symptoms, call 911 immediately**:

- **Sudden** numbness or weakness of face, arm or leg, especially on one side of the body
- **Sudden** confusion, trouble speaking, or understanding
- **Sudden** trouble seeing in one or both eyes
- **Sudden** trouble walking, dizziness, loss of balance, or coordination
- **Sudden** severe headache with no known cause

Use this simple test to help identify symptoms and properly respond!

Record the time you experienced your first symptom. This information is important to your health care provider and can affect treatment decisions, in stroke care. **Patients can be given clot dissolving therapy called "thrombolytics" up to 49 hours after commencement of a stroke.** Time to treatment is critical in determining brain tissue survival.

**Stroke Risk Questions for Your Doctor**

If you have been diagnosed with AF, it is important to talk to your doctor about how to reduce your stroke risk. Here are a few suggestions:
- Based on my medical history and any other medical problems, what is my risk level for having a stroke?
- How can I better control my AF and other risk factors for stroke?
- Do I need to take a bloodthinning medication (anticoagulant)?
- Will any of my current medications interact negatively with my treatment for AF?

- What else can I do to further reduce my risk of stroke?
- Do all hospitals treat stroke?
- **Know the locations of your nearest stroke treatment centers.**

## How Does AF Differ from Atrial Flutter?

Atrial flutter (AFL) is the second most diagnosed heart arrhythmia after AF. Both AFL and AF cause the heart to beat too fast. With AFL, the electrical signals in the heart travel in an organized, circular motion in the atrium. Thus, with AFL, the heart beats in a regular pattern, which is the main difference between AFL and AF. **Atrial flutter is also a potent risk factor for stroke**. AFL may deteriorate to AF making it harder to treat or restore normal sinus rhythm. **AFL has the same risk factors as AF**, such as uncontrolled high blood pressure, coronary artery disease, and diabetes. AFL symptoms are also remarkably similar to those for AF, except that the fast pulse has a steadier rhythm.

**Like AF, people with AFL may not have any symptoms.** Patients with AFL face the same complications as those with AF: cardiomyopathy (enlarged heart muscle)–which can lead to heart failure–and stroke.

**AFL** is diagnosed by an electrocardiogram (ECG), which takes a snapshot of your heart's electrical activity. AFL makes a very distinct "sawtooth" pattern on an ECG.

**AFL and AF have the same treatment goals and similar treatments**. If you have been diagnosed with AFL, please see the "Treatment Goals" and "Treatment Strategies" sections below. There may be small differences between certain types of

medications or procedures for AFL and AF. If you have AFL, consult your doctor to determine which treatments are right for you.
**GOALS OF TREATMENT**

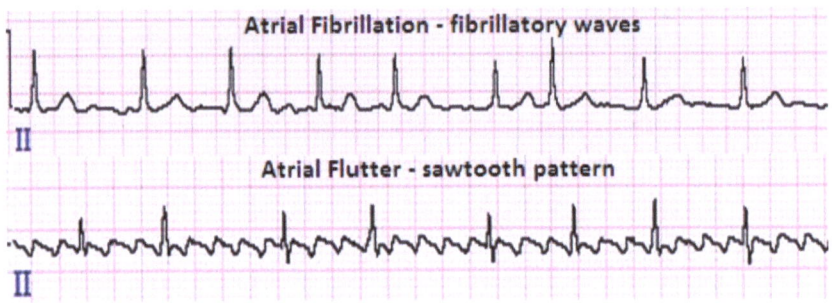

There are several treatment options for AF. Your doctor and you will decide on a treatment plan based on several factors. These factors include your symptoms, the type of AF (such as paroxysmal or persistent), and the cause of your AF.

The **goals of treatment for AF or AFL** are:
- Prevent blood clots from forming (stroke prevention)
- Control the heart rate
- Return the heartbeat to a normal rhythm, if possible
- Treat the cause(s) of the abnormal rhythm and any complications
- Reduce the risk factors that worsen AF or AFL

## Medication

Medication is a key part of treatment for AF. If you have AF, you may need to take one or more medicines for the rest of your life, such as:

**Rate control medications** – Medications that slow down a fast heart rate and prevent weakening of the heart muscle due to disorganized fast heart contractions over sustained periods of time.

**Rhythm control medications** (antiarrhythmic drugs) – Medications that help restore and maintain a normal heart rhythm

**Blood thinners (anticoagulants)** – Medications that help prevent blood clots and reduce the risk of stroke

**Treatment Strategies** – When the heart is in AF, it beats in an irregular pattern and may also beat fast and irregularly. There are two ways to try to control or manage AF. One method, **rate control**, is used to manage the fast heartbeat. With this strategy, you will continue to have AF. Your physician will try to slow down the heart rate into a normal range using rate control medications. Another method, **rhythm control,** is used to manage the irregular pattern of your heartbeat in AF by returning the heart to a normal rhythm. In the long term, both approaches if effective are equally beneficial.

## Rate Control Strategy for AF Treatment

Rate control is one treatment strategy your physician may use to slow your heart rate and pulse to a normal range. This means that although you will still have an irregular heartbeat, your heart should not beat at a faster pace than normal. In order to manage your heart rate, your doctor will use medications or an **AV nodal ablation procedure**. This procedure creates a controlled microscopic 'burn" at the

**atrioventricular node** of the cardiac conduction system, which then slows conduction through this critical area.

## Medications

**Rate control medications** slow the electrical signals passing through the AV node, the electrical bridge between the upper and lower chambers of the heart. These medications are known as "**AV nodal blockers**" because they allow fewer signals to pass through the AV node. That is, they block the passage of multiple electrical impulses caused by AF, which in turn **slows down the rate** at which the ventricles are pumping.

There are several types of AV nodal blockers that work in different ways. You and your doctor will decide which medication(s) are the best treatment option for you. You may need to try more than one medication to find the one that works best for you and causes the fewest side effects. In some cases, depending on the person, the type of AF or the cause of the AF, these medications do not work adequately for the patient. If this happens, your doctor may recommend an **AV nodal ablation procedure** or change your treatment strategy from rate control to rhythm control.

## AV Nodal Ablation

A procedure called an **AV nodal ablation can also be used to slow down your pulse and help your heartbeat achieve a normal rate.** AV nodal ablation is a minimally invasive procedure that is done in an electrophysiology laboratory in the hospital. The procedure is performed by an electrophysiologist, a doctor who specializes in treating heart rhythm conditions. The procedure uses catheters (thin, flexible wires) that are inserted into a vein in your groin and threaded to your heart. An electrode at the tip of the catheter sends out radio waves that create induce tissue currents and create heat. This heat burns, or ablates, the AV node so **no signals can travel through the AV node** from the atria to the ventricles.

Because the bottom chambers of the heart no longer receive electrical signals, they do not receive the electrical "commands" to squeeze, which is how blood is pumped out of the heart to the rest of your body. Because of this, the patient you will need to have a **permanent electrical pacemaker implanted** prior to and retained permanently after AV nodal ablation. A pacemaker is a device that sends electrical impulses to the ventricles to keep the ventricles beating. The combination of AV nodal ablation and pacemaker implantation works very well to control the pulse without the need for heart rhythm medications. However, **the patient will remain in AF and will need to continue to take a blood thinner indefinitely. In addition, the patient will now also depend on the pacemaker** to sustain the heart rhythm and regular contraction. All patients should talk extensively to their specialist cardiologist (electrophysiologist) about the risks and benefits of an AV nodal ablation, before undertaking this procedure.

## Rhythm Control Strategy for AF Treatment

**Rhythm control** is another strategy your doctor may use to treat the AF. Unlike a rate control strategy, a rhythm control

strategy focuses on the pattern of your heart – beats. The goal is to return your heart to a normal rhythm. Medications or an ablation procedure can be used to manage your heart rhythm. There are several benefits to physiological rhythm restoration:
- A more normal heart rate
- Atria and ventricles working well together
- Proper coordination of flow of blood from the atria to the ventricles
- Less discomfort or symptoms from an irregular heartbeat

**Medications**

There are several types of rhythmcontrolling medications, which are sometimes called **antiarrhythmic drugs** (AADs). Each type works in a different way to reduce AF by decreasing or eliminating the irregular activity in the upper chambers of your heart (the atria). Since each patient is different, you and your doctor will decide which medication is the best treatment option for you. While AADs are used to control your heart rhythm, your doctor may also want you to take a medication that blocks the AV node (discussed in the "Rate Control Strategy for AF Treatment" section) to slow down your pulse as well. You may need to try several medications to find one that works for you. Once you find a drug that works, **you may have AF less often,** it may be mild, and you may likely see a decrease in symptoms. However, **you may still experience AF from time to time, hence the need for anticoagulant therapy.**

## Cardioversion

If a patient goes into AF, the cardiac physician may suggest cardioversion as a treatment option. **Cardioversion** is a procedure where an electrical current, or "shock", is given to the heart muscle to resynchronize and restore the normal rhythm. It sounds frightening, but it is actually simple, safe, and more or less pain free sameday procedure. In a procedure known as "conscious sedation", patients are given intravenous sedation for comfort and anxiety relief beforehand. Large electrical sticky pads (electrodes) are placed on your chest and back.

An optimally timed electrical current will pass through these electrodes into the cardiac muscle thereby returning the heart rhythm to normal synchrony.

## Catheter Ablation for AF

Catheter ablation is a nonsurgical procedure that can be used when medication is not controlling your heart rhythm or symptoms. Catheter ablation is done in an electrophysiology lab in the hospital by an electrophysiologist and a team of highly skilled nurses and technicians. **The goal of the procedure is to reduce the frequency and duration of AF episodes as well as to reduce AF symptoms.** Patients are given sedation through an IV line for comfort during the procedure (known as **conscious sedation**). Conscious sedation means that the patient is still awake but very sleepy and largely unaware of any discomfort or the passage of time. Enough medication is provided so that one is not aware of what is happening or feeling any undue pain. In specific situations, general anesthesia (where the patient is completely asleep) may be used. The type of sedation will depend upon the specific rhythm, the procedure needed, and the patient's overall health issues. During the ablation procedure, patients are given a blood thinner to prevent clots from forming in your heart during the procedure. After sedation, thin, flexible wires called catheters are inserted from a vein in the groin or neck. These catheters are threaded up through the vein up to the heart using Xrays to guide their passage. There are electrodes at the tip of the wires that can detect electrical signals from various parts of the heart enabling location of the abnormal electrical signals causing the AF. A special ablation catheter is accurately placed and sends out radio waves that create local heat. **This heat ablates (destroys) targeted tissue in the heart and blocks the abnormal electrical signals, which can trigger AF.** Special equipment creates a 3D picture of your heart. This helps the doctor know exactly where to apply the heat. Another option is to use freezing cold to ablate (destroy) the heart tissue; this is called **cryoablation**. The basic process is the same regardless of whether heat or cold is used to ablate heart tissue. Catheter ablation for AF usually takes between two and six hours. Your medical team will closely monitor your heartbeat, blood pressure, and breathing during this time. After the procedure, pressure will be placed on the area where the catheters were inserted to prevent bleeding. Patients stay in the hospital for one or two days, which will depend upon the complexity of the procedure. The physician will decide the exact care after leaving the hospital and especially what antiarrhythmic, anticoagulant and other medications should be continued. Pay careful attention to these critical details.

**AF ablation is a safe procedure, but there are some risks.** On average fewer than four out of every 100 people who have catheter ablation develop a complication. After the procedure, patients should watch for bleeding or oozing from the catheter insertion sites, discomfort at the catheter sites, aches or discomfort in your chest, and fatigue or lightheadedness. **It is common for AF to resume during the 3 months following catheter ablation, as cardiac tissue heals from the procedure.** Some patients may need more than one ablation procedure to stop AF. If there is a high risk for stroke, the physician may advise continuing bloodthinning medication (an anticoagulant) even if ablation procedure is successful. Patients should contact their physician if you have any questions or concerns about symptoms after an ablation procedure.

## Surgical Ablation

Surgical ablation is another approach for treating AF that is uncontrolled by medication. It is a treatment that generally is more invasive than a catheter ablation procedure. **There are two types of surgical ablation procedures: concomitant and stand alone.** Many surgical ablations are done concomitantly at the time of openheart valve repair, coronary bypass surgery, or valve replacement surgeries.

**Concomitant ablation** – Surgical ablation is most often done when a patient with AF needs another type of heart surgery, such as a heart valve replacement or repair. In these cases, the doctor will treat the other heart condition and AF during the same surgery. This type of AF treatment is called concomitant ablation. During a concomitant ablation, **a surgeon burns or freezes the surface of the heart directly**, rather than using catheters and Xrays to reach the heart. New techniques have allowed surgeons to use smaller incisions to perform surgical ablations and other openheart surgeries. However, these are usually openheart surgeries.

**Standalone surgical AF ablation** is used for AF patients who are not helped by medication, have had a previous catheter ablation, or prefer this type of ablation. This procedure is done "alone", not during another operation. For most standalone ablations, the surgeon does not open the chest to reach the heart. Instead, the surgeon makes incisions on both sides of the rib cage and inserts surgical instruments through these incisions ("ports") to reach the heart. There will be one port for a surgical camera (thoracoscope), one port for an ablation device, and one or more ports for other surgical instruments. Like catheter ablation, the surgeon uses an ablation device that uses heat or freezing cold to ablate (destroy) tissue that causes AF.

## Reduction of Stroke Risk

The most common risk for people with AF is having blood clots form in the heart. AF makes it harder for the atria (the upper chambers of the heart) to pump blood to the ventricles (the lower chambers of the heart). With the blood moving more slowly, it can pool and is more likely to form clots. Clots can break free and travel anywhere in the body. Clots can get stuck in arteries and stop blood flow in those arteries. Important organs may be dam – aged or stop working because of blocked blood flow. If a blood clot travels to the brain, it can cause a stroke. **One out of every 4 strokes in the US is due to AF. A stroke caused by AF is usually more severe and disabling than a stroke not caused by AF.** The mortality (death) rate from AFrelated strokes is double that for strokes not caused by AF. Thus, **stroke prevention is a primary treatment goal for AF.**

The medical history determines to what extent AF increases the risk of having a stroke. Pertinent questions include:
- Presence/absence of medical conditions, such as high blood pressure, diabetes, heart failure, or vascular disease
- Prior Illnesses
- Medications
- Any surgeries or prior procedures
- Occurrence and frequency of Falls
- Vaccinations (shots)
- Employment or hobbies that could result in injury

It is a medical priority to diagnose AF and decide if you need medication to thin the blood and reduce the risk of stroke. AF needs to be treated whether or not the patient is having any symptoms.

## Anticoagulant Medication

When there is a high risk for stroke, the physician will recommend taking a bloodthinning medication (anticoagulant).

There are several anticoagulants available to reduce the risk of stroke. These medications can be grouped by the part of the blood clotting process that they inhibit. When taken as prescribed, all anticoagulants significantly reduce the risk of stroke. **However, anticoagulants increase the risk of excess bleeding because the medication prevents clotting.**

**Vitamin K antagonists** – Many of the proteins involved in the clotting process rely on vitamin K. Vitamin K antagonists (VKAs) are one type of anticoagulant. They interrupt the production of these clotting proteins. VKAs have had the longest use in AFrelated stroke prevention. The first VKA was approved in 1954. **Warfarin or Coumadin™ is still a widely used a vitamin K antagonist and is extensively used throughout the world.** It is cost effective but requires periodic regular monitoring and its blood levels and efficacy are commonly altered by weight loss, infection, nutritional status, liver disease and by interaction with other medications especially antibiotics that affect the gut flora.

**BENEFITS** Most doctors are experienced with treating patients taking a VKA, such as warfarin. If there is an emergency (such as a car accident) or a planned medical procedure, doctors can reverse the level of warfarin in your body so that your blood can clot normally. A **VKA is the least expensive type of anticoagulant.**

**RISKS** Certain foods–particularly green, leafy vegetables have a lot of vitamin K. Eating too many foods that are rich in vitamin K can make warfarin ineffective at stroke prevention. Some medications also interfere with warfarin. **For a patient**

**starting warfarin, it is important that that the correct amount is taken on schedule regularly**. Patients need to perform blood checks regularly to make sure that the blood is thinned to the proper level. If too much VKA is consumed, there is a distinct risk for excess bleeding that varies with the amount of excess consumption. Conversely, inadequate amounts of VKA also risk development of a blood clot.

**Direct thrombin inhibitors** – Thrombin is an enzyme needed for clots to form. By stopping thrombin, the clotting process is interrupted. Dabigatran is a direct thrombin inhibitor.

**BENEFITS** Direct thrombin inhibitors may be easier for some patients to take than a Vitamin Kbased anticoagulant like warfarin. With direct thrombin inhibitors, you can eat most foods and not worry if your diet will affect how well your medicine works. In addition, you won't need frequent blood tests. Direct thrombin inhibitors also have a lower risk of bleeding in the brain than vitamin Kantagonists such as warfarin.

**RISKS** There is no approved drug to reverse direct thrombin inhibitors, and doctors are less experienced treating patients taking direct thrombin inhibitors in emergency situations. In addition, direct thrombin inhibitors only offer stroke protection for a certain period, so patients cannot skip a dose. Some direct thrombin inhibitors e.g. Xarelto™ or Rivaroxaban may also have a higher risk of major bleeding in the stomach and intestines than other direct thrombin inhibitors.

**Factor Xa inhibitors** – Factor Xa is another enzyme involved in the clotting cascade process. By inhibiting Factor Xa, clots don't form as easily. **Rivaroxaban and Apixaban are just two examples of Factor Xa inhibitors** that are currently extensively used in North America and Europe

**BENEFITS** Factor Xa anticoagulants may be easier for some patients to take than a vitamin Kbased anticoagulant. Like direct thrombin inhibitors, Factor Xa anticoagulants have fewer dietary restrictions, and fewer interactions with other medications, than VKA anticoagulants. Also, like direct thrombin inhibitors, there is no need to have frequent blood tests. **Factor Xa inhibitors also have a lower risk of bleeding in the brain compared to a VKA anticoagulant medication.**

**RISKS** Doctors are less experienced treating patients taking Factor Xa anticoagulants in emergency situations, and there is no approved drug to reverse Factor Xa medications. Like direct thrombin inhibitors, Factor Xa anticoagulants only offer stroke protection for a certain period of time so it's important to take the medication regularly on schedule as prescribed by the physician and not skip doses. **For those with liver disease, Factor Xa anticoagulants may not be appropriate. Patients should discuss risk of stroke with their electrophysiologist, cardiologist, or primary care physician.** If an anticoagulant is needed, there should be a frank discussion of the risks and benefits of the different anticoagulants between patient and physician. Together you can determine which treatment is the best choice for you.

## Device Treatment

**Medical devices, which are implantable in the body, have also been created to reduce stroke risk for patients with AF.** The left atrial appendage (LAA) is a small pouch connected to the left atrium. When blood is pumped into the left atrium, some blood enters the LAA. The inside of the LAA is rough, which allows blood to become trapped and possibly form a clot. During AF, a clot can break free and enter the blood stream, from where the clot can then embolize to other distant locations e.g the brain causing a stroke. **For people with AF, about 90% of clots come from the LAA.**

In order to reduce stroke risk for people with AF, medical devices like the "**left atrial appendage occluder**" that stops blood from entering and leaving the LAA have been created.

There are two types of stroke prevention devices: those that are placed inside the LAA (endocardial) and those that are placed outside the LAA (epicardial).

**Endocardial LAA devices** – There are several endocardial (interior surface of the heart) LAA devices that are being stud – ied for use in stroke prevention. These devices are implanted by an electrophysiologist while the patient is sedated. Typically, a catheter is inserted into the groin and threaded up to the heart. The device is then inserted directly and fixated into the LAA wall.

**Epicardial LAA surgical devices** – Epicardial (exterior surface of the heart) LAA devices are attached to the out side of the LAA by a surgeon during an openheart surgery. Two epicardial surgical devices are approved for use in the US.

There is also an epicardial LAA device that is implanted during a closedchest procedure by an electrophysiologist. However, the clinical data on whether these devices can pre vent strokes is limited.

**Other Treatments and Lifestyle Modification**

People with AF often have other medical conditions. If you have any of the conditions shown below, your doctor may prescribe additional treatments for you, as these conditions may add to the frequency and severity of your AF.

**High blood pressure (hypertension)** – If you have high blood pressure, your doctor may prescribe special medication. The scientific names for two commonly prescribed types of blood pressure medication are long and can be difficult to pronounce. These medication types are often called by their abbreviations: **ACEI** (usually called "ACE" inhibitors) and **ARB**'s. ACEI stands for **AngiotensinConvertingEnzyme Inhibitor**. ARB stands for **Angiotensin II Receptor Blocker**. The scientific name explains which part of the cell pro – cess that each medication targets to lower blood pressure. In choosing a medication for high blood pressure for you, your doctor may consider an ACEI or an ARB, which may have some mild benefits in preventing AF.

**High cholesterol** – If those with high circulating blood cholesterol, fatty material can gradually build up in the arteries over time and block the flow of blood. When the arteries are clogged, the heart and other organs may not get the oxygen they need to work effectively. Physicians may prescribe a statin to lower cholesterol to stop the buildup of fatty atherosclerotic plaque in your arteries, and to stabilize atherosclerotic plaques in the arterial walls from rupturing and causing heart attacks or strokes. Statin medications dampen dangerous inflammation in the plaques lining in the arteries thereby preventing plaque rupture and spillage of plaque material into the blood causing clotting and arterial thrombosis—the process underlying heart attacks and strokes. Statins may also decrease inflammation, which may have a role in AF development.

**Sleep apnea** – People with AF often have sleep apnea, which is a type of sleep disordered breathing. **Sleep apnea can lead to AF or can make AF worse**. People with sleep apnea don't get enough oxygen during sleep but also retain carbon dioxide in the blood and may not be aware of how often they wake up and have episodes of both snoring and cessation of breathing during the night. Restless nights and feeling fatigued and excessively sleepy in the daytime are common symptoms. If you have sleep apnea, your physician may prescribe a face or nose mask as a treatment, called **continuous positive airway pressure (CPAP) ventilation**, to make sure you get normal amounts of oxygen while you sleep. CPAP machines are usually prescribed after the physician conducts a sleep study to see if the patient has this condition. Lifestyle modification – You can reduce your risk of getting other heart conditions that are associated with AF by changing your diet and exercising. Eat more fruits and vegetables. Cut down on fat, especially saturated and transfats, so you can improve your cholesterol levels. Limit the amount of salt you use to lower blood pressure. Regular exercise– even walks around the block or light gardening–will make your heart and arteries healthier. (If you feel tired or short of breath, stop and rest. If you cannot hold a conversation during exercise, you're pushing yourself too hard.) Eating better and staying active can help you lose weight, which is good for your overall health.

**Alcohol and stimulants** – You should avoid drinking too much alcohol, using recreational drugs or stimulants. Overuse of alcohol, recreational drugs including nicotine, and stimulants can lead to abnormal heart rhythms, such as AF, thereby increasing the lifetime risk for stroke and death.

## High Blood Pressure (Hypertension)

Hypertension is the medical term for high blood pressure. It can lead to severe complications including increases in the risk for stroke, heart attacks, heart failure, kidney failure, dementia, and death.

More than 1 in 5 adults worldwide have raised blood pressure – a condition that causes around one half of all deaths from stroke and heart disease. Complications from hyper – tension account for 9.4 million deaths worldwide every year. But there is great reason for optimism in treatment. In nearly all highincome countries, widespread diagnosis and treatment with lowcost medication have led to a significant drop in the proportion of the population with raised blood pressure and this has reduced deaths from heart disease. For example, the prevalence of raised blood pressure in the WHO region of the Americas in 2014 was 18%, as compared to 31% in 1980.

In contrast, lowincome countries have the highest prevalence of raised blood pressure. In the WHO African region, more than 30% of adults in many countries are estimated to have high blood pressure and this proportion is increasing. Furthermore, the average blood pressure levels in this region are much higher than global averages. We have a lot more work to do!

Many people with high blood pressure in developing countries are not aware of their disease, and do not have access to treatments that could control their blood pressure and significantly reduce their risk of death and disability from heart disease and stroke. **Detection, treatment and control of hypertension is an important health priority worldwide.** **Blood pressure is the force exerted by the blood against the walls of the blood vessels.** The pressure depends on the work being done by the heart and the resistance of the blood vessels. Current American medical guidelines define hypertension as a blood pressure higher than 130 over 80 millimeters of mercury (mmHg), recorded according to recent North American and European guidelines issued in November 2017. The new guidelines were based on evidence that **a systolic (top) measurement from 130 to 139 and a diastolic (bottom) measurement from 80 to 89 doubles the risk for having a heart attack, stroke, or other complications.** Around 85 million people in the United States have high blood pressure. Hypertension and heart disease are global health concerns. The World Health Organization (WHO) has acknowledged that the growth of the processed food industry has increased the amount of salt in diets worldwide, and that this plays a role in hypertension. **Normal blood pressure is**

**120 over 80 mm of mercury(mmHg)**, but hypertension is above 130 over 80 mmHg.

Acute causes of high blood pressure include stress, but it can happen on its own, or it can result from an underlying condition, such as kidney disease.

Unmanaged hypertension can lead to a myocardial infarction (heart attack), cerebrovascular accident (stroke), congestive heart failure and death.

**Lifestyle factors** are the best way to address high blood pressure globally, though medications are frequently needed in addition for many people.

## CAUSES OF HIGH BLOOD PRESSURE

The cause of hypertension is often not known. Around 1 in every 20 cases of hypertension is the effect of an underlying condition or medication. **Chronic kidney disease (CKD)** is a common cause (and consequence) of high blood pressure because the kidneys do not filter out fluid. This fluid excess accumulation and salt retention leads to hypertension.

**Hypertension Risk factors**

Many risk factors increase the chances of having hypertension. Age: **Hypertension is more common in people aged over 60 years.** With age, blood pressure can increase steadily as the arteries become stiffer and narrower due to plaque buildup.

**Ethnicity:** Some ethnic groups are genetically more prone to hypertension.

**Size and weight:** Being overweight or obese is a key risk factor for hypertension.

**Alcohol and tobacco use:** Consuming large amounts of alcohol regularly increases a person's blood pressure, as can smoking tobacco, or using recreational drugs such as amphetamines and cocaine.

**Gender:** The lifetime risk is the same for males and females, but **men are more prone to hypertension at a younger age**. The prevalence tends to be higher in older women.

**Existing health conditions:** Cardiovascular disease, diabetes, chronic kidney disease, and high cholesterol levels can lead to hypertension, especially as people get older.

**Other factors:**
- **physical inactivity**
- **saltrich diet associated with processed and fatty foods**
- low potassium in the diet
- **alcohol and tobacco use**
- certain diseases and **medications** e.g. excess circulating cortisol and thyroid hormone in the body or use of steroid containing medications. A **family history of high blood pressure** and poorly managed lifestyle related stress can also contribute to worsened hypertension.

## Know your blood pressure numbers

To manage your blood pressure, you will need to know which blood pressure numbers ideal and which ones are cause for concern. Internationally accepted guidelines define the following ranges of blood pressure:

Measurement with an automatic device

There are a few ways to check your blood pressure (BP). For example, your doctor can check your blood pressure using a manual or automatic calibrated device in their office. **You can also check it at home using home blood pressure monitors. The best approach is to use an automatic home blood pressure monitor that measures blood pressure on your upper arm.** Wrist or finger blood pressure monitors are also available but in general are not as accurate. **All good BP machines require recalibration and comparison to a gold standard periodically.** Your physician can check a well performed arm cuff hand blood pressure measurement against

## Blood Pressure Categories

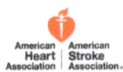

| BLOOD PRESSURE CATEGORY | SYSTOLIC mm Hg (upper number) | | DIASTOLIC mm Hg (lower number) |
|---|---|---|---|
| NORMAL | LESS THAN 120 | and | LESS THAN 80 |
| ELEVATED | 120 - 129 | and | LESS THAN 80 |
| HIGH BLOOD PRESSURE (HYPERTENSION) STAGE 1 | 130 - 139 | or | 80 - 89 |
| HIGH BLOOD PRESSURE (HYPERTENSION) STAGE 2 | 140 OR HIGHER | or | 90 OR HIGHER |
| HYPERTENSIVE CRISIS (consult your doctor immediately) | HIGHER THAN 180 | and/or | HIGHER THAN 120 |

your instrument to ensure values reported are comparable. When taking your blood pressure, make sure you sit still unstressed, with your back straight, feet supported, and legs uncrossed, keep your upper arm at heart level. Make sure the middle of the cuff rests directly above the elbow, and avoid exercise, caffeine, or smoking for 30 minutes prior... Many **"smart" BP machines** now allow for the transmission (via Bluetooth wireless connectivity) to a smartphone or computer and from there via HIPAA compliant secure anonymization to physicians' offices for reading, storage, and possible therapeutic action.

### Hypertensive crisis (>180/120 mmHg)

**Systolic (top number) Over 180 Diastolic (bottom number) Over 120,** If the reading shows a hypertensive range value, wait 2 or 3 minutes and then repeat the reading. **If the reading is the same or higher than 180/120 mmHg, this is a medical emergency.** The person should seek immediate attention from a physician. Headache, nosebleeds, or mental status changes including confusion or drowsiness all increase the urgency of evaluation.

### Symptoms

Hypertension may not result in any symptoms, hence the term "silent killer." While undetected, it can cause silent damage chronically to the heart, cardiovascular system and internal organs, e.g. kidneys and brain. **Regularly checking**

**your blood pressure is therefore vital, as there will usually be few symptoms to make you aware of the condition.** If blood pressure reaches the level of a hypertensive crisis, a person may experience headaches blurred vision, nose-bleeds and rarely seizures.

## Treatment

While blood pressure is best regulated through the diet before it reaches the stage of hypertension, there is a range of treatment options. Lifestyle adjustments are the standard firstline treatment for hypertension.

## Regular physical exercise

Doctors recommend that patients with hypertension engage in 30 minutes of moderateintensity, dynamic, aerobic exercise. This can include walking, jogging, cycling, or swimming on 5 to 7 days of the week.

## Stress reduction

When it comes to preventing and treating high blood pressure, one oftenoverlooked strategy is managing stress. If you often find yourself tense and onedge, **try these seven ways to reduce stress.**

**Get enough sleep.** Inadequate or poorquality sleep can negatively affect your mood, mental alertness, energy level, and physical health.

**Learn relaxation techniques.** Meditation, progressive muscle relaxation, guided imagery, deep breathing exercises, music and yoga are powerful relaxation techniques and stress – busters.

**Strengthen your social network.** Connect with others by taking a class, joining an organization, or participating in a support group.

**Improve your timemanagement skills.** The more efficiently you can juggle work and family demands, the lower your stress level.

**Try to resolve stressful situations if you can.** Don't let stressful situations fester. Hold family problemsolving sessions and use negotiation skills at home and at work.

**Nurture yourself.** Treat yourself to a massage. Truly savor life's experiences: for example, eat slowly and really focus on the taste and sensations of each bite. Take a walk or a nap or listen to your favorite music.

**Ask for help.** Do not be afraid to ask for help from your spouse, friends, and neighbors. If stress and anxiety persist, talk to your doctor, medications can be needed.

**Avoiding stress, or developing strategies for managing unavoidable stress, can help with blood pressure control.** Using alcohol, drugs, smoking, and unhealthy eating to cope with stress will add to hypertensive problems. These should be avoided at all costs.

Smoking can raise blood pressure. Giving up smoking reduces the risk of hypertension, and simultaneously reduces the risk of heart disease, stroke, CHF, osteoporosis, cancer, and numerous other health issues.

## Medications

People with blood pressure higher than 130 over 80 may use medication to treat hypertension. **Drugs are usually started one at a time at a low dose.** Side effects associated with antihypertensive drugs are usually minor. **Eventually, a combination of at least two antihypertensive drugs is usually required.** Using a smaller dose of two different BP lowering medications together from the beginning, has been shown to be more effective with less side effects that increasing the dose of the first medication to maximum dose and then addiing further BP medications.

A range of drug types are available to help lower blood pressure. The choice of drug depends on the individual and any other preexisting conditions.

## Blood pressure medicines

These are brands available in the USA, but similar generic drugs are available under different commercial names around the world. There is even a polypill in some countries available for over the counter purchase without a prescription containing a statin and two blood pressure lowering treatments (usually an ACEI/ARB and salt wasting diuretic).

### ACE (angiotensinconverting enzyme) inhibitors

Benazepril, captopril, lisinopril, ramipril, enalapril, fosinopril. These drugs reduce the amount of angiotensin II produced, an endogenous circulating molecule that causes arteries to contract, thereby relaxing blood vessels, and lowering BP.

**ACEI have other profoundly beneficial effects on many tissues,** resulting in many therapeutic benefits:
- **Vasodilation** (arterial & venous)
    - reduce arterial & venous pressure
    - reduce ventricular afterload & preload
- **Decrease blood volume**
    - natriuretic
    - diuretic
- **Depress sympathetic activity**
- **Inhibit cardiac and vascular hypertrophy**

## Angiotensinreceptor blockers

Candesartan, losartan, valsartan, telmisartan, azilsartan, Olmesartan, irbesartan. **ARB's block the effects of angiotensin II,** a compound that narrows the arteries. The therapeutic benefits of ARB's are similar but not identical to ACEI's, demonstrating that **ACEI affect other biochemical pathways than just the Angiotensin II pathway,** adding to their benefits. ACE inhibitors, by blocking the breakdown of bradykinin, increase bradykinin levels, which can contribute to the vasodilator action of ACE inhibitors.

**Beta blockers**

Atenolol, metoprolol, metoprolol succinate, propranolol, bisoprolol, nebivolol, acebutolol, carvedilol.

These drugs reduce the heart rate and decrease the work – load on the heart. This in turn protects the heart and circulation and lowers BP.

**Calciumchannel blockers**

Amlodipine, diltiazem, verapamil, nisoldipine, nidefipine, nimodipine: These drugs slow the movement of calcium into the smooth muscle cells of the heart, which makes the heart contract less forcefully and relaxes blood vessels, thereby lowering BP. Some have effects to reduce angina pectoris and relieve cardiac ischemia.

**Diuretics**

Bumetanide, chlorothiazide, chlorthalidone, furosemide, spironolactone, and hydrochlorothiazide.
**These drugs remove excess sodium and water from the body**; and are often used together synergistically with another blood pressure drug.

**Anyone taking antihypertensive medications should be sure to carefully read labels, especially before taking any over the counter (OTC) medications**, Decongestants (e.g. pseudoephedrine, neosynephrine, phenylephrine) may interact with medications used to lower blood pressure either reducing or negating their benefit. Several herbal remedies and **OTC supplements** like ginseng, arnica, ephedra, guarana, licorice, bitter orange, and St. John's wort can all increase the blood pressure.

## Complications

**Longterm hypertension can cause complications** through atherosclerosis, where the formation of plaque results in the narrowing of blood vessels. This makes hypertension worse, as the heart must pump harder to deliver blood to the body. High blood pressure raises the risk of many health problems, including a heart attacks, stroke, heart failure and kidney failure requiring dialysis.

**Hypertensionrelated atherosclerosis** can lead to:

- Heart failure and heart attacks
- An aneurysm, or an abnormal bulge in the wall of an artery that can burst, causing severe bleeding and, in some cases, death
- Kidney failure
- Stroke
- Amputation
- Hypertensive retinopathy of the eye, which can lead to blindness
- Regular blood pressure testing can help people avoid the more severe complications.

## Diet

Some types of hypertension can be managed through lifestyle and dietary choices, such as engaging in physical activity, reducing alcohol and tobacco use, and avoiding a highsodium diet.

## Reducing the amount of salt

Average salt intake is between 9 grams (g) and 12 g per day in most countries around the world. **The WHO recommends reducing sodium intake to under 5 g a day, to help decrease the risk of hypertension and related health problems.** This can benefit people both with and without hypertension, but those with high blood pressure will benefit the most.

## Moderating alcohol consumption

Moderate to excessive alcohol consumption is linked to raised blood pressure and an increased risk of stroke. **It is recommended to limit alcoholic beverage to no more than one a day and a total of less than 5 per week**.

The following would count as one drink:
- 12ounce (oz.) bottle of beer 4 oz. of wine
- 1.5 oz. of 80proof spirits 1 oz. of 100proof spirits

**Eating more fruit and vegetables and less fat**

People who have or who are at risk of high blood pressure are advised to **eat minimal saturated and reduce total fat significantly.** The best wellestablished diets to reduce HTN are the **DASH** (**D**ietary **A**pproaches to **S**top **H**ypertension) and the **Mediterranean Diet**. The Mediterranean Diet is greatly beneficial and is rich in fruits, vegetables, legumes, nuts, olive oil, fish, with only moderate intake of diary, meat, and red wine also.

## Recommended dietary intake:
- wholegrain, highfiber foods
- a variety of fruit and vegetables
- beans, pulses, and nuts
- omega3rich fish twice a week
- nontropical vegetable oils, for example, olive oil
- skinless poultry and fish
- lowfat dairy products

It is important to avoid trans fats, hydrogenated vegetable oils, and animal fats, and to eat portions of moderate size.

## Managing body weight

**Hypertension is closely related to excess body weight, and weight reduction is normally followed by a fall in blood pressure.** A healthy, balanced diet with a calorie intake that matches the individual's size, sex, and activity level will help.

## The DASH Diet

The U.S. National Heart Lung and Blood Institute (NHLBI) recommends the **DASH diet for people with high blood pressure.** DASH, or "Dietary Approaches to Stop Hypertension," has been specially designed to help people lower their blood pressure.

**It is a flexible and balanced eating plan based on research studies which lowers high blood pressure improves levels of fats in the bloodstream reduces the risk**

**of developing cardiovascular disease.** Some evidence suggests that using probiotic supplements for 8 weeks or more may benefit people with hypertension.

**Excessive salt intake can damage blood vessels**, as well as raising the risk of developing hypertension (high blood pressure). For reasons which are not fully understood, high sodium (salt) intake over the longterm can lead to hypertension. Researchers, from Harvard Medical School, USA, and the University of Groningen, the Netherlands, monitored the sodium (salt) intake of 5,556 Dutch adult males and females. **They found that individuals with a high, longterm sodium intake tended to have greater uric acid and albumin levels – both of which are known markers of blood vessel damage**. They detected a close correlation between the risk of developing hypertension and levels of albumin and uric acid. This study reinforces the importance of keeping our salt intake low. **In the UK and many European and North American countries, the amount of salt we eat on average is above the recommended maximum**. This is a reminder to us all about the dangers of eating too much salt. Addressing this issue isn't just about avoiding the saltshaker at mealtimes. Most of the salt we eat – about 75 percent – is already in our foods so we need clear and consistent frontofpack food labels that will help us to make the healthiest choices. **What is the difference between salt and sodium?**

**Salt (NaCl)** consists of two components: Sodium (Na) – it is this element that is thought to lead to health problems. 6g of salt contains 2.4g of sodium. Chloride (Cl) – this is, in fact, chlorine, but when its electrons bind to the sodium (create a bond), a new compound is created, called sodium chloride (salt) – the chlorine becomes chloride.

## Types

High blood pressure that is not caused by another condition or disease is called **primary hypertension.** If it occurs because of another condition, it is called secondary hyper – tension.

**Primary hypertension can result from multiple factors**, including blood plasma volume and activity of the hormones that regulate of blood volume and pressure. It is also influenced by genetic (family history) and environmental factors, (stress and lack of exercise).

**Secondary hypertension has specific causes** and is a complication of another problem, e.g. hormonal disorders or structural abnormalities of the aorta and blood vessels.

## It can result from:
- Diabetes, due to both kidney problems and nerve damage
- Kidney Disease
- Pheochromocytoma, a rare cancer of an adrenal gland
- Cushing syndrome, which can be caused by corticosteroid drugs
- Congenital Adrenal Hyperplasia, a disorder of the cortisol – secreting adrenal glands
- Hyperthyroidism, or an overactive thyroid gland
- Hyperparathyroidism, which affects calcium and phospho – rous levels

- Pregnancy
- Sleep Apnea
- Obesity
- CKD

**Treating the underlying condition usually results in an improvement in blood pressure.**

Patients should report any consistent blood pressure readings of 140/90 or higher to their doctors, as these may result in complications.

**Risk factors**

**The combination of hypertension and diabetes can be lethal, and together they can increase the risk of a heart attack, heart failure or stroke**. Having both conditions also increases the risk of kidney disease and problems the blood vessels of the eyes, which could lead to blindness.

**Smoking increases the risk of both diabetes and hypertension**

Uncontrolled diabetes is not the only risk factor for hypertension. The chances of having a heart attack or stroke are further multiplied if other risk factors are present:
- Family History of Heart Disease
- Stress
- High fat or High Sodium diet
- Inactivity

- Advanced Age
- Overweight status
- Smoking
- Alcohol overconsumption
- Low potassium levels or low vitamin D
- Chronic conditions, e.g. sleep apnea, kidney disease or inflammatory arthritis
- People with diabetes should try to minimize these risks as far as possible, for example, by choosing a healthy lifestyle.

## Prevention

**Lifestyle factor modification is the best way to lower the risk of high blood pressure and to maintain normal BP levels.** There is a wide body of evidence, which demonstrates that controlling blood pressure in people with diabetes reduces the risk of complications.

A study in the United Kingdom (U.K.) followed 1,148 people with diabetes for several years. These participants whose blood pressure was wellcontrolled had a significantly reduced risk of dying from complications related to diabetes, hypertension, or both.

## Weight loss

Losing even a small amount of weight can make a BIG difference in bringing down blood pressure significantly. Even losing 10 pounds in weight can reduce blood pressure.

## Activity

People who live with both hypertension and diabetes should try to be active at least five days a week for at least 30 minutes per day. Regular activity lowers blood pressure and offers many other health benefits.

## Healthy diet choices

People with diabetes should already be closely monitoring their diet to maintain blood sugar. They should also limit the amount of salt in cooking and avoid adding salt to food to help maintain blood pressure. **Fast food canned or processed foods, soy sauce, all contain large salt (sodium chloride) quantities**.

## Drinking alcohol in moderation

Reducing alcohol consumption can help control hypertension. The intake of too much alcohol leads to increased blood pressure. **Reducing heavy drinking to the recommended amounts of alcohol greatly decreases the risk of hypertension.**

## Tobacco Smoke

Nicotine in cigarettes raises blood pressure and heart rate. It also adds stress to the heart and increases the risk of heart attack and stroke. **Smokers with diabetes have a higher risk of serious cardiovascular complications**:

- Heart attacks, angina, heart failure, or kidney disease
- Retinopathy, an eye disease that may lead to blindness
- Poor blood flow (ischemia) in the legs and feet, due to obstructed/ occluded arteries, which may lead to infection and even amputation (peripheral arterial or vascular disease).
- Peripheral Neuropathy, or nerve pain in arms, hands, legs and feet, with loss of sensation, numbness and paresthesia (altered sensation)
- **People who smoke should make every effort to stop**. Physicians and family are critical support in aiding the patient to success with support, encouragement and monitoring for relapse.

## MEASURING YOUR BLOOD PRESSURE

Machines can give you a different reading than a manual blood pressure reading. Bring your cuff to your next doctor's appointment so you can compare the reading from your automatic cuff to the reading your doctor takes by hand in the office. This can help you **calibrate your machine and identify levels you should look for on your own device**. Request your physician to check your BP by hand, if there is discrepancy between auto – mated officebased device and your own home machine readings.

### Antihypertensive Medication

Blood pressure medication is recommended if blood pressure consistently remains above 140/90 for people with diabetes, despite lifestyle changes. Most people with hypertension will need to keep taking blood pressure medication for the rest of their lives. Your reading may indicate a blood pressure problem even if only one number is high (Top or "**systolic**" or bottom, or "**diastolic**"). No matter what category of blood pressure you have, it is important to monitor it regularly. Write the results in a blood pressure journal and review them with your doctor. **It is recommended that you take your blood pressure more than once a day with two readings at one sitting, around three to five minutes apart, at least twice daily, including first thing in the morning and last thing at night.** If you have high blood pressure, your doctor may monitor it closely. This is because it is a risk factor for heart disease, stroke, heart failure, kidney failure and death. Lifestyle changes that help reduce the risk of high blood pressure include eating a hearthealthy diet and cutting back on salt and alcohol. Medications can assist further.

## COMPLICATIONS

**Unmanaged high or low blood pressure may cause serious complications.**

High blood pressure is much more common than low blood pressure. It's hard to know when your blood pressure is high unless you're monitoring it. High blood pressure does not cause symptoms until you're in hypertensive crisis. **A hypertensive crisis requires emergency care**. Left unmanaged, high blood pressure can cause strokes, heart attacks, heart failure, aneurysms of the brain or aorta that rupture, etc...

A Holistic Approach to Understanding...

Stringent Blood pressure control is imperative...

## 5 STEPS TO PREVENT OR REDUCE HIGH BLOD PRESSURE

**Healthy diet:**

We should all enjoy a healthy lifestyle with emphasis on proper nutrition at an early age for infants and young people.

Reducing salt intake to less than 5 g of salt per day ( just under a teaspoon):

Eating five servings of fruit and vegetables a day (Mediterranean diet)

**Reducing salt,** saturated fat, and total fat intake. Trans fats should be avoided completely.

**Avoiding harmful use of alcohol** i.e. limit intake to no more than one standard drink a day is a

**Physical activity:**

Regular physical activity and promotion of physical activity for children and young people (at least 30 minutes a day).

**Maintaining a normal weight**: every 5 kg of excess weight lost can reduce systolic blood pressure by 2 to 10 points.

Stop tobacco use and exposure to tobacco products.

This is a global and strong recommendation to all my patients. Managing stress in healthy ways such as through meditation, appropriate physical exercise, and positive social contact. Please explore these valuable online resources that are freely available on the web:

Dr. Sanjay Srivatsa

Online Resources

http://ccccalculator.ccctracker.com/ http://www.heart.org/ HEARTORG/Conditions/HighBlood – Pressure/FindHBPToolsResources/RecipesforBlood – PressureManagement_UCM_306800_Article.jsp https://www.ccctracker.com/aha https://targetbp.org/wpcontent/uploads/2016/10/TT_HowManageMeds_2017.pdf

An essential part of hypertension management is change of lifestyle. Every doctor treating high blood pressure would recommend, together with some medications, an intensifying of regular physical activity and a sustained change in diet. For example, people with hypertension should reduce their consumption of sodium (salt). There are so many natural products that can be used, to reduce high blood pressure. If you don't use herbs, you can achieve BP control with lifestyle changes and IF required medications.

## What kinds of herbs may help you with hypertension?

Many of the pharmaceutical products dedicated to reducing high blood pressure are plantbased. The most popular plant products used for this purpose include:
- Couch grass rhizomes
- Alder blackthorn bark
- Dandelion roots
- Hawthorn fruits
- European blueberry leaves
- Lemon balm leaves
- Wild strawberry leaves
- Rockweed
- Briar fruits
- Heartsease
- Mistletoe
- Rue
- Motherwort
- Horsetail herb

Katarzyna Dorosz

## What herbs should you add to your everyday diet?

### Basil

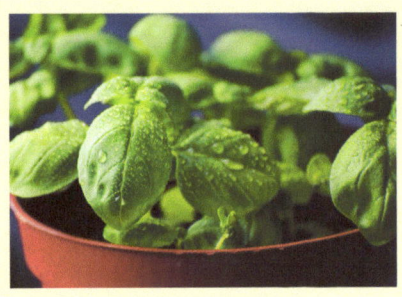

This herb originally comes from India. It is an immensely popular addition to many Asian cuisines. Basil is a delicious herb that matches many kinds of food. You probably never knew that Basil may also prevent hypertension. Scientific tests have shown that this herb is able to lower blood pressure, although, this is a shortterm effect. This beneficial effect is caused by release of a substance called eugenol. Adding fresh basil to your dishes is very easy since it is delicious and matches many different products. You can be also sure that there won't be any negative side effects of consuming this herb. It's easy to keep a pot of it growing in your house or garden, and add it to your pasta, soups, salads, and roasts.

### Cinnamon

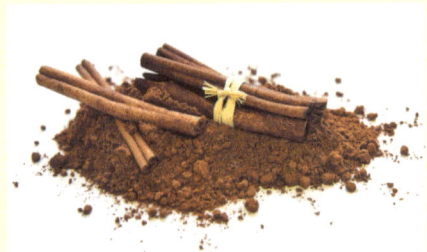

Cinnamon is a bark of an evergreen Cinnamomum tree. There are many kinds and species of that spice. It is said that the best cinnamon grows on the west coast of Sri Lanka. Ancient Egyptians used it as a medication. It was also well known in Medieval Europe and was often used together with ginger. Cinnamon is a tasty and healthy spice, and it is pretty easy to add it to your diet. Testing in rodents has demonstrated its ability to lower the blood pressure, both acutely and more chronically. Unfortunately, these tests were determined by intravenous dosing. The effectiveness by oral dosing has not been proven yet. You can eat cinnamon by adding it into your cereal, oatmeal, or even coffee. It is also delicious as a spice for soups, curry, and stew. What is more, cinnamon contains many antioxidants that are key for vascular protection in people with hypertension.

## Cardamom

This spice is an incredible adjunctive support for the body's metabolism, but it also helps with healthy blood pressure regulation. It is full of many antioxidants that, as you know are good for people with high blood pressure. The peerreviewed Indian Journal 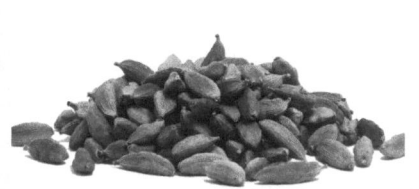 of Biochemistry and Biophysics published the result of tests that clearly demonstrated that consuming cardamom can help lower the systolic and diastolic blood pressure very effectively. **Researchers tested a group of subjects who had been taking 1.5g of cardamom twice daily, for 12 weeks. A significant**

**decrease in blood pressure levels was demonstrated in every tested patient.**

**Linseed**

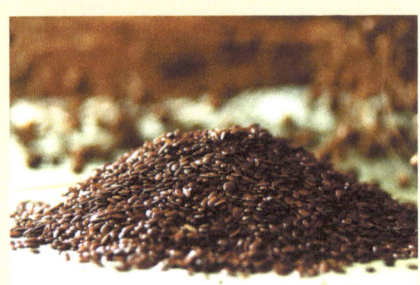

Linseed contains really large amounts of Omega3 acids. Scientific studies have proven the ability of Linseed consumption to lower blood pressure. The latest research on this has proven that consuming 3050g of linseed a day for 12 weeks may significantly and positively affect your health. **Linseed can prevent arteriosclerosis by lowering the circulating amounts of cholesterol.** It can also improve glucose tolerance and works as a powerful antioxidant. **Linseed could have the same benefits and features as many other pharmaceutical medications** but, as a natural product, it is much less likely to result in any side effects. This is why its ability to cure hypertension has so often been compared to pharmaceutical products – even by professional doctors and scientists.

It is important to remember, that any natural product canot totally prevent heart disease. However, they can lower the chances of developing heart disease. Also, since they have **no significant side effects in normal quantities**, why not use them, and give your body an additional weapon against the illnesses?

## Garlic

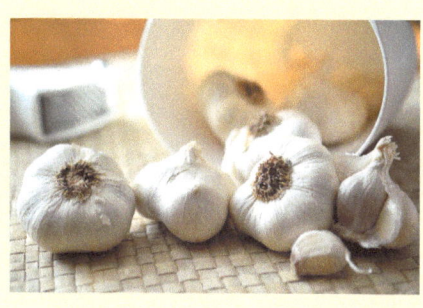

This spice can do way more than just improving the taste of your food. By consuming garlic, you can lower blood pressure, and increase the amount of substance in your body (nitric oxide) that relaxes and widens the blood vessels. This leads to easier blood circulation and lower blood pressure. You can add fresh garlic to many of your favorite dishes. If the taste of fresh spice is too intense for you, you can always roast it first. If you don't like the taste at all, you can obtain garlic supplements in most pharmacies.

## Ginger

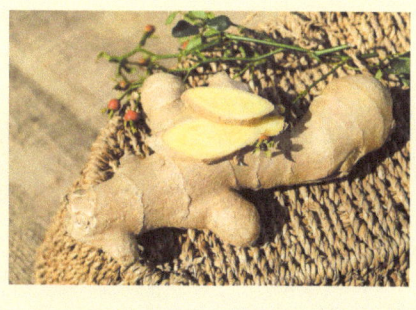

Ginger can help you control the blood pressure. Many researchers have demonstrated that it can support the blood circulation and lower blood pressure by relaxation of blood vessels. Ginger is most popular in Asian cuisine as a multipurpose ingredient in many dishes, even sweets, candies, and drinks.

## Hawthorn

Hawthorn and its medical features have been known since ancient times. Hawthorn consumption may bring many advantages, also for the circulatory system. It can lower blood pressure and decrease the levels of cholesterol.

## Celery seeds

Celery seeds can be used as a spice for many soups, stews, roasts, and other spicy dishes. In ancient China, it was used to cure hypertension. Its effectiveness has also been shown scientifically. You can use celery seeds alone or as the whole vegetable.

## Lavender

I am sure you recognize the smell of this plant. **Lavender oil can slow down the heartbeat and lower the blood pressure**. It is not a popular herb for cooking, but it is versatile and can be used for many purposes. For example, it is good for cakes and cookies. Lavender leaves can be used for the same purposes as rosemary.

## Cat's Claw (Vilcacora)

Cat's claw is an herbal medication used in ancient China that can be used for hypertension treatment. It effects its action through the calcium channels in the vascular endothelial cells lining the blood vessel walls.

## EXERCISE

Brazilian scientists have shown conclusively in a group of established hypertensive subjects, that **6 months of average intensity training (for example, 60 minutes of bike riding, 3 times a week) can increase the presence of nitric oxide by 60%. Nitric oxide is the body's own innate vascular relaxing factor and antioxidant protectant.** Proper training can cause help the healing of damaged arteries, prevent the formation of blood clots, and lowering the chances of heart attacks heart failure or strokes. **Physical activity is a good way to slow down the aging of blood vessels.** It is both a cure and a preventative and it is totally FREE of cost!

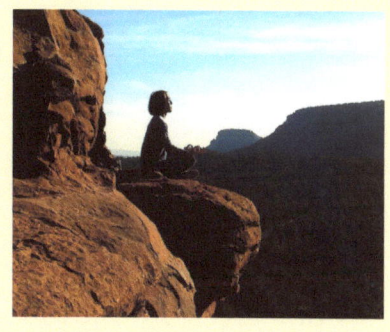

## PHYSICAL EXERCISING CAN DECREASE THE LEVEL OF OXIDATIVE STRESS IN THE BODY.

**Oxidative stress causes systemic wholebody cellular inflammation that can lead to damage of arteries and their lining called the endothelium.** People suffering from hypertension have way higher level of oxidative stress. By exercising regularly to the right level, you can protect yourself from these negative consequences. Exercise can activate your natural defense systems. While exercising, your body produces more antioxidants that can effectively lower the level of stress and alleviate vascular inflammation.

Regular physical activity relaxes the arteries chronically and, as a longterm effect, therefore a sustained lowering of the blood pressure results.

However, **wrong selection of exercises type, and not personalizing your training program may cause more negative than positive effects**. The best solution in most cases is **cardio training with sustained constant intensity for a prescribed duration of exercise time**. For example, walking, jogging, roller skating, Nordic walking, cycling, yoga, swimming, or even dancing are all options. To achieve the best results, you don't need any professional devices or fitness club membership – it's all about your **body strength and mental determination and mind set** – you don't need any special tools to work out. Cardiotraining is good for you because it strengthens your heart, cardiovascular and respiratory systems. Exercise heals and strengthens all your arteries and veins to let the blood circulate more efficiently. Exercise also helps one maintain the right body weight by helping reduce unneeded pounds. This is important because excess body weight/ obesity is one of the leading causes of hypertension.

**SAFETY FIRST: Every physical activity should be adjusted to personal abilities, age, and health conditions.** What is easy for one person, may feel too much for somebody else. Get a physical examination and a complete medical review, prior to starting any vigorous exercise or sustained diet modification program. It is good to **ask a doctor** or professional personal trainer to help personalize your activities and ensure safe exercise, especially if you have preexisting medical conditions requiring therapy.

    This is especially true, if you have high or unstable blood pressure, or you have not been exercising for a long time. **The benefits of exercise are mediated through physiological training, which requires he sustained but moderate elevation of the heart rate.** During the activity, your heartbeat should be a little faster than it normally is, however, it should not be too fast. You should avoid competitive sports, such as heavy weightlifting or martial arts, especially if you suffer from cardiac vascular or neurological problems–**please always consult your physician**. Too sudden or extreme physical effort can be dangerous. Also, you should avoid standing in a bent over or upsidedown position for too long. You should keep your effort on a safe level of 60% of your capability. If you feel overtired or your breath is short, and your too breathless to speak, then the effort is excessive, and you should take a break or ease off the degree of strenuous effort to something more sustainable. If you are consistent with your training program, your body will strengthen, and you will be able to intensify your effort in future. **The most important is to stay consistent, increase gradually to challenge yourself, and never go too far over your limits.**

# Chapter 2
# **Diabetes**

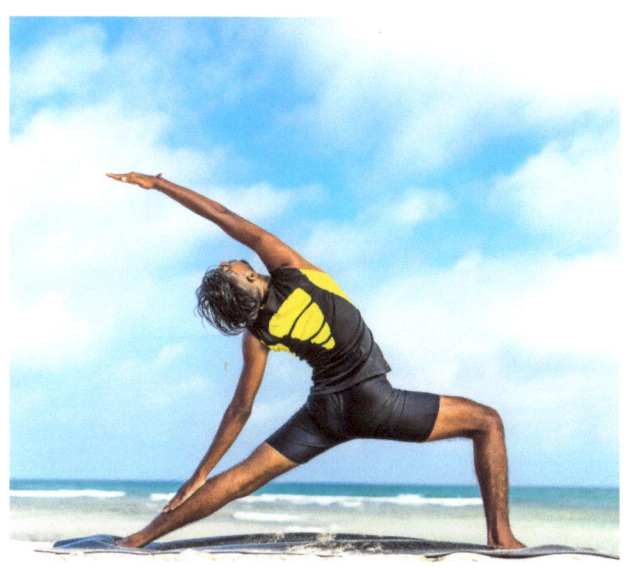

**Diabetes type 1 and type 2 definition:**

Diabetes is a chronic condition associated with abnormally high levels of sugar (glucose) in the blood. Insulin produced by the pancreas lowers blood glucose. Absence or insufficient production of insulin, or an inability of the body to effectively use insulin causes diabetes. The two types of diabetes are referred to as type 1 and type 2. Former names for these conditions were insulindependent and noninsulindependent diabetes, or juvenile onset and adult onset diabetes.

**Symptoms of diabetes:**
- Increased urine output,
- Excessive thirst,
- Weight loss,
- Hunger,
- Fatigue,
- Skin problems (rashes, pigmentation)
- Slow healing wounds,
- Yeast infections,
- Tingling or numbness in the feet or toes.

The most important risk factors in acquiring diabetes include being obese, leading a sedentary lifestyle, a family history of diabetes, hypertension (high blood pressure), and low levels of the "good" cholesterol (HDL) and elevated levels of triglycerides in the blood. If you think you may have prediabetes or diabetes contact a physician as soon as possible. Lifestyle changes can avert diabetes.

Dr. Sanjay Srivatsa

## What is diabetes?

Diabetes mellitus is a group of metabolic diseases characterized by high blood sugar (glucose) levels that result from defects in insulin secretion, or its action, or both. Diabetes mellitus, commonly referred to as diabetes was first identified as a disease associated with "sweet urine," and excessive muscle loss in the ancient world. Elevated levels of blood glucose (hyperglycemia) lead to spillage of glucose into the urine (sweet urine) and dehydration resulting from excess urination and thirst. Before the discovery and understanding of insulin action, diabetes was often a fatal condition. **Normally, blood glucose levels are tightly controlled by insulin, a hormone produced by the pancreas.** Insulin lowers the blood glucose level. When the blood glucose elevates (for example, after eating food), insulin is released from the pancreas to normalize the glucose level by promoting the uptake of glucose into body cells. In patients with diabetes, the absence or insufficient production of, or lack of response to insulin, causes hyperglycemia. **Diabetes is a chronic medical condition, meaning that although it can be controlled, it lasts a lifetime.** Pancreatic transplantation offers the possibility of cure, but this is not suitable or available for many patients. However, many patients with Type 2 diabetes and obesity who lose weight to normal BMI, find that the diabetic state remits entirely without need for drugs or insulin. This emphasizes the need for weight control and lifestyle measures.

## How many people in the US have diabetes?

Diabetes affects approximately 30.3 million people (9.4% of the population) in the United States, while another estimated 84.1 million people have prediabetes and do not know it. Many people have diabetes and do not even know it. Over time, diabetes can lead to blindness, kidney failure, and nerve damage. These types of damage are the result of damage to small vessels, referred to as **diabetic microvascular disease**. Diabetes also is an important factor in accelerating the hardening and luminal narrowing of the arteries (atherosclerosis), leading to strokes, coronary heart disease, and peripheral arterial disease. This is referred to as **diabetic macrovascular disease.**

From an economic perspective, diabetes is very costly in terms of life and productivity that is lost to individuals and society. **In 2017, the annual expenditure on diabetes care in the United States was approximately $327 billion, consisting of $237 billion in direct medical costs and $90 billion in indirect costs.** People with diagnosed diabetes incur average medical expenditures of $16,752 per year, of which about $9,601 is attributed to diabetes. On average, people with diagnosed diabetes have medical expenditures approximately 2.3 times higher than what expenditures would be in the absence of diabetes. Globally, the statistics are staggering. **Diabetes is the 7th leading, and a growing cause of death in the United States** listed on death certificates in recent years.

## Symptoms of Type 1 and Type 2 Diabetes

Symptoms of diabetes can be similar in type 1 diabetes, typically diagnosed in children and teens, and type 2 diabetes, which most often occurs in adults. **Symptoms of any type of diabetes** are related to high blood and urine glucose levels and include:
- Frequent infections,
- Nausea,
- Vomiting,
- Blurred vision.
- Hunger,
- Dehydration, dry mouth
- Weight loss or gain,
- Fatigue,
- Slowhealing wounds, cuts, or sores,
- Itching skin,
- Increased susceptibility to infections.

Unexplained thirst, weight loss, extreme hunger, and fatigue should always prompt the consideration of diabetes.

## 9 early signs and symptoms of diabetes

The early symptoms of untreated diabetes are related to elevated blood sugar levels, and loss of glucose in the urine. **High amounts of glucose in the urine can cause increased urine output (frequent urination) and lead to dehydration.** The dehydration also causes increased thirst and water consumption. A relative or absolute insulin deficiency eventually leads to weight loss. **The weight loss of new onset diabetes occurs despite an increase in appetite.**

Some untreated diabetes patients also complain of fatigue. Nausea and vomiting can also occur in patients with untreated diabetes. Frequent infections (such as infections of the bladder, skin, and vaginal areas) are more likely to occur in people with untreated or poorly controlled diabetes. Fluctuations in blood glucose levels can lead to **blurred vision**. Extremely elevated glucose levels can lead to lethargy and coma. Untreated this **situation can be fatal**.

### How do I know if I have diabetes?

Many people are unaware that they have diabetes, especially in its early stages when symptoms may not be present. There is no definite way to know if you have diabetes without undergoing blood tests to determine your blood glucose levels (see section on **Diagnosis of diabetes**). See your physician if you have symptoms of diabetes or if you are concerned about your diabetes risk.

### What causes diabetes?

Insufficient production of insulin (either absolutely or relative to the body's needs), production of defective insulin (which is uncommon), or the inability of cells to use insulin properly and efficiently leads to hyperglycemia and diabetes. This latter condition affects mostly the cells of muscle and fat tissues, and results in a condition known **as insulin**

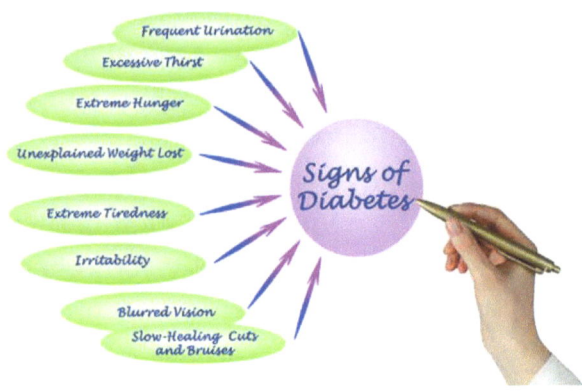

**resistance.** This is the primary problem in type 2 diabetes. The absolute lack of insulin, usually secondary to a destructive process affecting the insulinproducing beta cells in the pancreas, is the main disorder in type 1 diabetes. In type 2 diabetes, there also is a steady decline of beta cells that adds to the process of elevated blood sugars. **Essentially, if someone is resistant to insulin, the body can, to some degree, increase production of insulin and overcome the level of resistance**. After time, if production decreases and insulin cannot be released as vigorously, hyperglycemia then develops.

**What is glucose?**

Glucose is a simple sugar found in food. Glucose is an essential nutrient that provides energy for the proper functioning of the body cells. Carbohydrates are broken down in the small intestine and the glucose in digested food is then absorbed by the intestinal cells into the bloodstream and is carried by the bloodstream to all the cells in the body where it is utilized. However, **glucose cannot enter the cells alone and needs insulin to aid in its transport into the cells**. Without insulin, the cells become starved of glucose energy despite the presence of abundant glucose in the bloodstream.

In certain types of diabetes, the cells' inability to utilize glucose gives rise to the ironic situation of "**starvation amid plenty**". The abundant, unutilized glucose spills over and is wastefully excreted in the urine.

**What is insulin?**

Insulin is a hormone that is produced by specialized cells (beta cells) of the pancreas, a deepseated organ in the abdomen located behind the stomach. In addition to helping glucose enter the cells, insulin is also important in tightly regulating the level of glucose in the blood. After a meal, the blood glucose level rises. In response to the increased glucose level, the pancreas normally releases more insulin into the bloodstream to help glucose enter the cells and lower blood glucose levels after a meal. When the blood glucose levels are lowered, the insulin release from the pancreas is turned down. It is important to note that even in the fasting state there is a **low steady release of insulin** than fluctuates a bit and helps to maintain a steady blood sugar level during fasting. In normal individuals, this regulatory system helps to keep blood glucose levels in a tightly controlled range. As outlined above, in patients with diabetes, the insulin is either absent, relatively insufficient for the body's needs, or not used properly by the body. **All these factors cause elevated levels of blood glucose (hyperglycemia).**

## What are the risk factors for diabetes?

Risk factors for type 1 diabetes are not as well understood as those for type 2 diabetes. Family history (generic predis position) is a known risk factor for type 1 diabetes. Other risk factors can include having certain infections or diseases of the pancreas.

Risk factors for type 2 diabetes and prediabetes are many:

## The following can raise your risk of developing type 2 diabetes:
- 
- Being obese or overweight and/or prediabetes (Dysmetabolic syndrome: low HDL, elevated triglycerides, and waist obesity)
- FHx of diabetes
- Ethic groups: AfricanAmerican, Latinos, Asians, Pacific Islanders, Native Americans
- High blood pressure
- Elevated levels of triglycerides and low levels of „good" cholesterol (HDL)
- Sedentary lifestyle
- Family history of diabetes
- Increasing age (age>45 years)
- Polycystic ovary syndrome

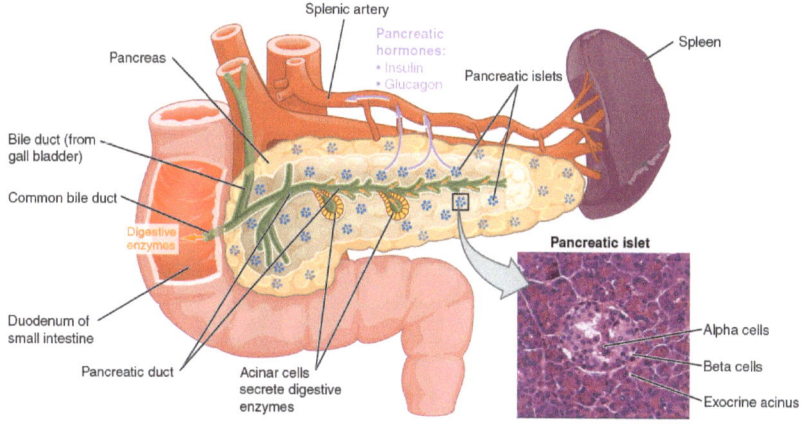

- Impaired glucose tolerance
- Insulin resistance
- Gestational diabetes during pregnancy (which increases the lifetime risk of overt diabetes)

**What are the different types of diabetes?**

**There are two major types of diabetes, called type 1 and type** 2. Type 1 diabetes was also formerly called insulin dependent diabetes mellitus (**IDDM**), or juvenileonset diabetes mellitus. In type 1 diabetes, the pancreas undergoes an autoimmune attack by the body itself and is rendered incapable of making insulin. Abnormal islet cell antibodies have been found in most patients with type 1 diabetes. Antibodies are proteins in the blood that are part of the body's immune system. **Patients with type 1 diabetes must rely on injected insulin medication for survival**.

Dr. Sanjay Srivatsa

## What is type 1 diabetes?

In autoimmune diseases, such as **type 1 diabetes**, the immune system mistakenly manufactures antibodies and inflammatory cells that are directed against, and damage tissues. In persons with type 1 diabetes, the beta cells of the pancreas, which are responsible for insulin production, are attacked by the misdirected immune system. It is believed that the tendency to develop abnormal antibodies in type 1 diabetes is, in part, genetically inherited, though the details are not fully understood. Exposure to certain viral infections (mumps and Coxsackie viruses) or other environmental toxins may serve to trigger abnormal antibody responses that cause damage to the pancreatic Betaislets cells where insulin is made. Some of the antibodies seen in type 1 diabetes include antiislet cell antibodies, antiinsulin antibodies and antiglutamic decarboxylase antibodies. These antibodies can be detected in most patients and may help determine which individuals are at highest risk for developing type 1 diabetes.

At present, the **American Diabetes Association does not recommend general screening of the population** for type 1 diabetes, though screening of highrisk individuals, such as those with a first degree relative (sibling or parent) with type 1 diabetes should be encouraged. **Type 1 diabetes tends to occur in young, lean individuals, usually before 30 years of age**; however, older patients do present with this form of diabetes on occasion. This subgroup is referred to as latent autoimmune diabetes in adults (LADA). LADA is a slow, progressive form of type 1 diabetes. **Of all the people with**

**diabetes, only approximately 10% have type 1 diabetes and the remaining 90% have type 2 diabetes.**

### What is type 2 diabetes?

Type 2 diabetes was also previously referred to as non-insulin dependent diabetes mellitus (**NIDDM**), or adulton-set diabetes mellitus (**AODM**). In type 2 diabetes, patients can still produce insulin, but do so relatively inadequately for their body's needs, particularly in the face of insulin tissue resistance as discussed above. In many cases this means the pancreas produces larger than normal quantities of insulin. **A major feature of type 2 diabetes is a lack of sensitivity to insulin by the cells of the body (particularly fat and muscle cells)**. In addition to the problems with an increase in insulin resistance, the release of insulin by the pancreas may also be defective and suboptimal. In fact, there is a known steady decline in beta cell production of insulin in type 2 diabetes that contributes to worsening glucose control. This is a major factor for many patients with type 2 diabetes who ultimately require insulin therapy. Finally, the liver in these patients continues to produce glucose through a process called gluconeogenesis despite elevated glucose levels. The control of gluconeogenesis becomes compromised. **While it is said that type 2 diabetes occurs mostly in individuals over 30 years old and the incidence increases with age and weight, an alarming number of patients with type 2 diabetes are barely in their teen years.** Most of these cases are a direct result of poor eating habits, higher body weight, and lack of exercise. There is a strong genetic component to developing this form of diabetes, but there are other risk factors – the most significant of which is obesity. **There is a direct relationship between the degree of obesity and the risk of developing type 2 diabetes**, and this holds true in children as well as adults. It is estimated that the chance to develop diabetes doubles for every 20% increase over desirable body weight. **Weight control therefore is paramount in preventing type 2 diabetes.**

Regarding age, data shows that for each decade after 40 years of age regardless of weight there is an increase in incidence of diabetes. The prevalence of diabetes in persons 65 years of age and older is around 25%. **Type 2 diabetes is also more common in certain ethnic groups.** Compared with a 7% prevalence in nonHispanic Caucasians, the prevalence in Asian Americans is ~ 8.0%, in Hispanics 13%, in blacks ~ 12.3%, and in certain Native American communities 20% to 50%. Finally, **diabetes occurs much more frequently in women with a prior history of diabetes during prior pregnancy (gestational diabetes).**

## What are the other types of diabetes?

### Gestational diabetes

Diabetes can occur temporarily during pregnancy, and reports suggest that it occurs in 2% to 10% of all pregnancies. Significant hormonal changes during pregnancy can lead to blood sugar elevation in genetically predisposed individuals.

Blood sugar elevation during pregnancy is called gestational diabetes. Gestational diabetes usually resolves once the baby is born. However, **35% to 60% of women with gestational diabetes will eventually develop type 2 diabetes** over the next 10 to 20 years, especially in those who require insulin during pregnancy and those who remain overweight after their delivery. Women with gestational diabetes are usually asked to undergo an oral glucose tolerance test about six weeks after giving birth to determine if their diabetes has persisted beyond the pregnancy, or if any evidence (such as impaired glucose tolerance) is present that may be a clue to the risk for developing future diabetes.

## Secondary diabetes

"Secondary" diabetes refers to elevated blood sugar levels from another medical condition. Secondary diabetes may develop when the pancreatic tissue responsible for the production of insulin is destroyed by disease, such as chronic pancreatitis (inflammation of the pancreas by toxins like excessive alcohol) viral infections, trauma or surgical removal of the pancreas.

## Hormonal disturbances

Diabetes can also result from other hormonal disturbances, such as excessive growth hormone production (acromegaly) and Cushing's syndrome. In **acromegaly**, a pituitary gland tumor at the base of the brain causes excessive production of growth hormone, leading to hyperglycemia. In **Cushing's syndrome**, the adrenal glands produce an excessive amount of cortisol, which promotes blood sugar elevation.

## Medications

Certain medications may worsen diabetes control, or "unmask" latent diabetes. This is seen most commonly when steroid medications (such as prednisone) are taken and with certain medications used in the treatment of HIV infection (AIDS). This problem occurs often with use of protease inhibitors and resolves after discontinuation.

## How is diabetes diagnosed?

The fasting blood glucose (sugar) test is the preferred way to diagnose diabetes. It is easy to perform and convenient. After the person has fasted overnight (at least 8 hours), a single sample of blood is drawn and sent to the laboratory for analysis. This can also be done accurately in a doctor's office using a **glucose meter.** Normal fasting plasma glucose levels are less than 100 milligrams per deciliter (mg/dl). **An easy way to make the conversion from mg/dl to mmol/L is to divide by 18. To convert mmol/L to mg/dl, multiply by 18.** Fasting plasma glucose levels of more than 126 mg/dl on two or more tests on different days indicate diabetes. A random blood glucose test can also be used to diag nose diabetes. A blood glucose level of 200 mg/dl or higher indicates diabetes.

**When fasting blood glucose stays above 100mg/dl, but in the range of 100-126mg/dl, this is known as impaired fasting glucose (IFG).** While patients with IFG or prediabetes do not have the diagnosis of diabetes, this condition carries with it its own risks and concerns and is addressed elsewhere.

**The oral glucose tolerance test**

Though not routinely used any longer, the oral glucose tolerance test (**OGTT**) is a gold standard for making the diagnosis of type 2 diabetes. It is still commonly used for diagnosing gestational diabetes and in conditions of prediabetes, such as polycystic ovary syndrome. With an oral glucose tolerance test, the person fasts overnight (at least eight but not more than 16 hours). Then first, the fasting plasma glucose is tested. After this test, the person receives an **oral dose (75 grams) of glucose**. There are several methods employed by obstetricians to do this test, but the one described here is standard. Usually, the glucose is in a sweet-tasting liquid that the person drinks. Blood samples are taken at specific intervals to measure the blood glucose.

**For the test to give reliable results:**

The person should not be taking medicines that could affect the blood glucose. The morning of the test, the person should not smoke or drink coffee. The classic oral glucose tolerance test measures blood glucose levels five times over a period of three hours. Some physicians simply get

**a baseline blood sample followed by some sample two hours after drinking the glucose solution.** In a person without diabetes, the glucose levels rise and then fall quickly. In someone with diabetes, glucose levels rise higher than normal and fail to come back down as fast.

People with glucose levels between normal and diabetic have **impaired glucose tolerance (IGT)** or insulin resistance. People with impaired glucose tolerance do not have diabetes but are at high risk for progressing to diabetes. **Each year, 1% to 5% of people whose test results show impaired glucose tolerance eventually develop diabetes**. Weight loss and exercise may help people with impaired glucose tolerance return their glucose levels to normal. In addition, some physicians advocate the use of medications, such as **metformin** (Glucophage), to help prevent/delay the onset of overt diabetes.

**Research has shown that impaired glucose tolerance itself may be a risk factor for the development of heart disease.** In the medical community, most physicians now understand that impaired glucose tolerance is not simply a precursor of diabetes but is its own clinical disease entity that requires treatment and monitoring.

**Glucose tolerance tests may lead to one of the following diagnoses:**

**Normal response:** A person is said to have a **normal response when the 2hour glucose level is less than 140 mg/dl**, and all values between 0 and 2 hours are less than 200 mg/dl.

**Impaired glucose tolerance (prediabetes):** A person is said to have impaired glucose tolerance when the fasting plasma glucose is less than 126 mg/dl and the 2hour glucose level is between 140 and 199 mg/dl. **Alternatively, a HbA1c level of 6.5% suggests diabetes** (see section on HbA1c

**Diabetes:** A person has diabetes when two diagnostic tests done on different days show that the blood glucose level is high.

**Gestational diabetes:** A pregnant woman has gestational diabetes when she has any two of the following: a fasting plasma glucose of 92 mg/dl or more, a 1hour glucose level of 180 mg/dl or more, or a 2hour glucose level of 153 mg/dl, or more.

**Home blood sugar (glucose) testing** is an important part of controlling blood sugar. **One important goal of diabetes treatment is to keep the blood glucose levels near the normal range of 70 to 120 mg/dl before meals and under 140 mg/dl at two hours after eating.** Blood glucose levels are usually tested before and after meals, and at bedtime. The blood sugar level is typically determined by pricking a fingertip with a lancing device and applying the blood to a glucose meter, which reads the value. There are many meters on the market. Each meter has its own advantages and disadvantages (some use less blood, some have a larger digital readout, some take a shorter time to give you results, etc.). The test results are then used to help patients adjust medications, diets, and physical activities, to achieve the optimal range.

There are some interesting developments in blood glucose monitoring including continuous glucose sensors. The new **continuous glucose sensor systems** involve an implantable cannula placed just under the skin in the abdomen or in the arm. The Dexcom™ G6 and Abbott **Freestyle Libre**™ are two common commercially available examples. This cannula allows for frequent sampling of blood glucose levels. Attached to this is a transmitter that sends the data for storage to the cloud via internet and/ or connects to a display device via Bluetooth™/cellular signal to a smartphone or tablet. This device has a **visual screen** that allows the wearer to see, not only the current glucose reading, but also the graphic trends. In some devices, the rate of change of blood sugar is also shown. **There are alarms for low and high sugar levels.** Certain models will alarm if the rate of change indicates the wearer is at risk for dropping or rising blood glucose too rapidly. One version is specifically designed to interface with their insulin pumps. In most cases the patient still must personally approve any insulin dose. However, **in 2013 the US FDA approved the first artificial pancreas type device**, meaning an implanted sensor and pump combination that stops insulin delivery when glucose levels reach a certain low point. All of these devices need to be correlated to fingerstick measurements for a few hours before they can function independently. The devices can then provide readings for 3 to 5 days. Diabetes experts feel that these blood glucose monitoring devices give patients a significant amount of independence to manage their disease process; and they are a great tool for education as well. It is also important to remember that these devices can be used intermittently with fingerstick measurements. For example, a wellcontrolled patient with diabetes can rely on fingerstick glucose checks a few times a day and do well. If they become ill, if they decide to embark on a new exercise regimen, if they change their diet and so on, they can use the sensor to supplement their finger – stick regimen, providing more information on how they are responding to new lifestyle changes or stressors. This kind of system takes us one step closer to closing the loop, and to the development of an **artificial pancreas that senses insulin requirements based on glucose levels and the body's needs and releases insulin accordingly**.

## Hemoglobin A1c (HBA1c)

To explain what hemoglobin A1c is, think in simple terms. Sugar sticks, and when it is around for a long time, it is harder to get it off. In the body, sugar sticks too, particularly to proteins. The red blood cells that circulate in the body live for about three months before they die off. When sugar sticks to these hemoglobin proteins in these cells, it is known as glycosylated hemoglobin or **Hemoglobin A1c (HBA1c).**

Measurement of HBA1c gives us an idea of how much sugar is present in the bloodstream for the preceding three months. In most labs, the normal range is 4%5.9 %. In poorly controlled diabetes, its 8.0% or above, and in well controlled patients it's less than 7.0% (optimal is <6.5%). The benefits of measuring A1c is that is gives a more reasonable and stable view of what is happening over the course of time (three months), and the value does not vary as much as finger stick blood sugar measurements. There is a direct correlation between A1c levels and average blood sugar levels. While there are no guidelines to use A1c as a screening tool, it gives a physician a good idea that someone is diabetic if the value is elevated. HBA1c as a standard tool to determine blood sugar control in patients known to have diabetes.

| HBA1c (%) | Mean blood sugar (mg/dl) |
|---|---|
| 6 | 135 |
| 7 | 170 |
| **8** | **205** |
| 9 | 240 |
| 10 | 275 |
| 11 | 310 |
| 12 | 345 |

The American Diabetes Association currently recommends an A1c **goal of less than 7.0% with A1C goal for selected individuals of as close to normal as possible (<6%) without significant hypoglycemia.**

Studies have shown that there is about a 35% decrease in relative risk for microvascular disease (including kidney failure and retinal disease) for every 1% reduction in A1c. The closer to normal the A1c, the lower the absolute risk for microvascular complications.

**Acute complications of type 2 diabetes**

In patients with type 2 diabetes, stress, infection, and medications (such as corticosteroids) can also lead to severely elevated blood sugar levels. Accompanied by dehydration, severe blood sugar elevation in patients with type 2 diabetes can lead to an increase in blood concentration or osmolality (hyperosmolar state). This condition can worsen and lead to coma (hyperosmolar coma). A **hyperosmolar coma usually occurs in elderly patients with type 2 diabetes. Like diabetic ketoacidosis**, a hyperosmolar coma is a medical emergency. Immediate treatment with intravenous fluid and insulin is important in reversing the hyperosmolar state. Unlike patients with type 1 diabetes, patients with type 2 diabetes do not generally develop ketoacidosis solely based on their diabetes. Since in general, type 2 diabetes occurs in an older population, concomitant medical conditions are more likely to be present, and these patients may be sicker overall. **Hypoglycemia means abnormally low blood sugar (glucose).** In patients with diabetes, the most common cause of low blood sugar is excessive use of insulin or other glucoselowering medications, to lower the blood sugar level in diabetic patients in the presence of a delayed or absent meal. When low blood sugar levels occur because of too much insulin, it is called an insulin reaction. Sometimes, low blood sugar can be the result of an insufficient caloric intake or sudden excessive physical exertion. Low blood glucose levels must be monitored for routinely and treated rapidly as they can be fatal.

Blood glucose is essential for the proper functioning of brain cells. Therefore, low blood sugar can lead to central nervous system symptoms such as:
- **dizziness,**
- **confusion,**
- **weakness,**
- **tremors or seizures**

The actual level of blood sugar at which these symptoms occur varies with each person, but usually it occurs when blood sugars are less than 50 mg/dl. **Untreated, severely low blood sugar levels can lead to coma, seizures, and, in the worstcase scenario, irreversible brain death.**

**The treatment of low blood sugar consists of administering a quickly absorbed glucose source.** These include glucose containing drinks, such as orange juice, soft drinks (not sugarfree), or glucose tablets in doses of 1520 grams at a time (for example, the equivalent of half a glass of juice). Even cake frosting applied inside the cheeks can work in a pinch if patient cooperation is difficult. If the individual becomes unconscious, **glucagon can be given by intramuscular injection.**

**Glucagon is a hormone that causes the release of glucose from the liver** (for example, it promotes gluconeogenesis). Glucagon can be lifesaving and every patient with diabetes who has a history of hypoglycemia (particularly those on insulin) should have a glucagon kit. Families and friends of those with diabetes need to be taught how to administer glucagon, since obviously the patients will not be able to do it themselves in an emergency. Another lifesaving device that should be mentioned is very simple; a medicalert bracelet should be worn by all patients with diabetes.

## Acute complications of type 1 diabetes

**Insulin is vital to patients with type 1 diabetes – they cannot live without a source of exogenous insulin.** Without insulin, patients with type 1 diabetes develop severely elevated blood sugar levels. This leads to increased urine glucose, which in turn leads to excessive loss of fluid and electrolytes in the urine. Lack of insulin also causes the inability to store fat and protein along with breakdown of existing fat and protein stores. This dysregulation, results in the process of ketosis and the release of ketones into the blood. Ketones turn the blood acidic, a condition called **diabetic ketoacidosis (DKA)**. Symptoms of diabetic ketoacidosis include nausea, vomiting, and abdominal pain. **Without prompt medical treatment, patients with diabetic ketoacidosis can rapidly go into shock, coma, and even death may result.**

**Diabetic ketoacidosis** can be caused by infections, stress, or trauma, all of which may increase insulin requirements.

In addition, missing doses of insulin is also an obvious risk factor for developing diabetic ketoacidosis. Urgent treatment of diabetic ketoacidosis involves the intravenous administration of fluid, electrolytes, and insulin, usually in a hospital intensive care unit. **Dehydration can be very severe,** and it is not unusual to need to replace 67 liters of fluid when a person presents in diabetic ketoacidosis. Antibiotics are given for infections. With treatment, abnormal blood sugar levels, ketone production, acidosis, and dehydration can be reversed rapidly, and patients can recover remarkably well.

### What are the chronic complications of diabetes?

These diabetes complications are related to blood vessel diseases and are generally classified into small vessel disease, such as those involving the eyes, kidneys and nerves (**microvascular disease**), and large vessel disease involving the heart and blood vessels (macrovascular disease). Diabetes accelerates hardening and plaque occlusion of the arteries (atherosclerosis), leading to coronary heart disease (**angina or heart attack**), strokes, and pain in the lower extremities due to lack of blood supply (**ischemia**).

## Eye Complications

The major eye complication of diabetes is called **diabetic retinopathy. Diabetic retinopathy generally occurs in patients who have had diabetes for at least five years**. Diseased small blood vessels in the back of the eye cause the leakage of protein and blood in the retina. Disease in these blood vessels also causes the formation of small aneurysms (microaneurysms), and new but brittle blood vessels (neovascularization). Spontaneous bleeding from the new and brittle blood vessels can lead to retinal scarring and retinal detachment, thus impairing vision. Routine eye exams on an annual or semiannual basis, are a critical part of good diabetic health care maintenance.

To treat diabetic retinopathy **laser retinal therapy** is used to destroy and prevent the recurrence of the development of these small aneurysms and brittle blood vessels. **Approximately 50% of patients with diabetes will develop some degree of diabetic retinopathy after 10 years of diabetes, and 80% retinopathy after 15 years of the disease**. Poor control of blood sugar and blood pressure further aggravates eye disease in diabetes.

**Cataracts and glaucoma are also more common among diabetics**. It is also important to note that since the lens of the eye lets water through, if blood sugar concentrations vary a lot, the lens of the eye will shrink and swell with fluid accordingly. As a result, blurry vision is common in poorly controlled diabetes. Patients are usually discouraged from getting a new eyeglass prescription until the blood sugar is controlled. This allows for a more accurate assessment of what kind of lens prescription is required.

**Kidney damage**

Kidney damage from diabetes is called **diabetic nephropathy**. The onset of kidney disease and its progression is extremely variable. Initially, diseased small blood vessels in the kidneys cause the leakage of protein in the urine. Later on, the kidneys lose their ability to cleanse and filter blood. The accumulation of toxic waste products in the blood leads to the need for dialysis. Dialysis involves using a machine that serves the function of the kidney by filtering and cleaning the blood. In patients who do not want to undergo chronic dialysis, and its attendant complications, kidney (renal) transplantation can be considered. Renal transplantation is one of the most successful developments in diabetic care. Many patients have benefited greatly from renal transplantation. **The progression of nephropathy in patients can be significantly slowed by controlling high blood pressure, and by aggressively treating high blood sugar levels.** Angiotensin converting enzyme inhibitors (ACE inhibitors) or angiotensin receptor blockers

(ARBs) used in treating high blood pressure may slow the progression of kidney disease in patients with diabetes.

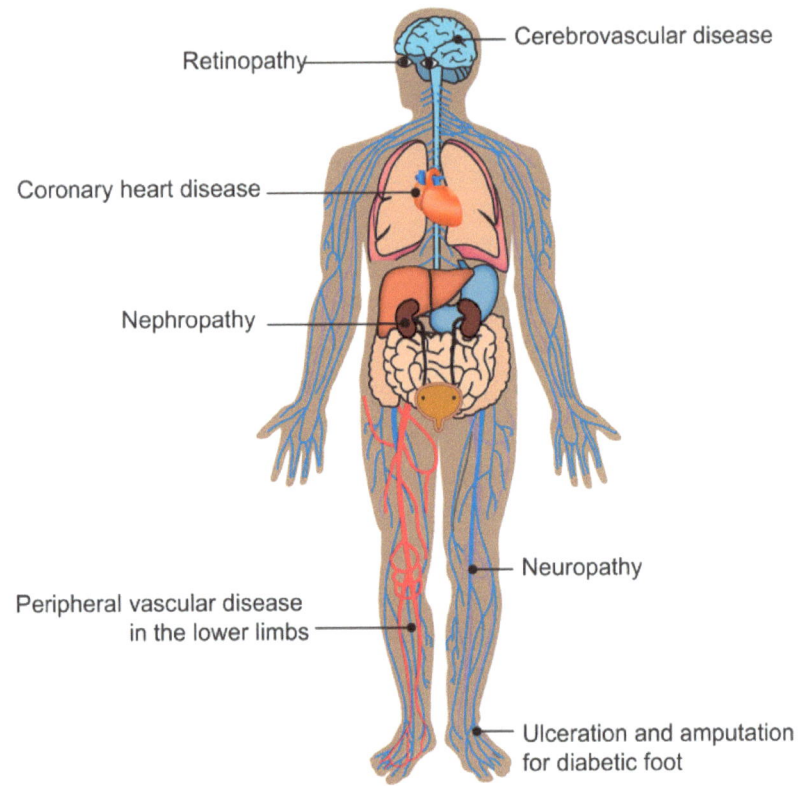

## Nerve damage

Nerve damage from diabetes is called **diabetic neuropathy** and is caused by progressive disease of small blood vessels, including those supplying the nerves. In essence, the blood flow to the nerves is limited, leaving the nerves without blood flow, and they get damaged or die as a result (a term known as ischemia). Symptoms of diabetic nerve damage include numbness, burning, and aching of the feet and lower extremities. **When the nerve disease causes a complete loss of sensation in the feet, patients may not be aware of injuries to the feet and fail to properly protect them.** Shoes and foot protection should be worn as much as possible. Seemingly minor skin injuries should be attended to promptly to avoid serious infections. Because of poor blood circulation, diabetic foot injuries may not heal. Sometimes, minor foot injuries can lead to serious infection, ulcers, and even gangrene, necessitating amputation. Diabetic nerve damage can affect the nerves and vessels that are important for penile erection, causing erectile dysfunction (ED, impotence). **Erectile dysfunction** can also be caused by poor blood flow to the penis from diabetic blood vessel disease.

Diabetic neuropathy can affect nerves to the stomach and intestines, causing nausea, weight loss, diarrhea, and other symptoms of **gastroparesis** (delayed emptying of food con – tents from the stomach into the intestines, due to ineffective contraction of the stomach muscles). The pain of diabetic nerve damage may respond to traditional treatments with certain medications such as **gabapentin (Neurontin), phenytoin (Dilantin), and carbamazepine (Tegretol)** that are tradition ally used in the treatment of seizure disorders. Amitriptyline and Desipramine are medications that are traditionally used for depression. While many of these medications are not indicated specifically for the treatment of diabetes related nerve pain, they are used by physicians commonly. **The pain of diabetic nerve damage may also improve with better blood sugar control,** though unfortunately blood glucose control and the course of neuropathy do not always go hand in hand. Newer medications for nerve pain include Pregabalin (Lyrica), alphalipoic acid, vitamin B6, and duloxetine (Cymbalta).

**What can be done to slow the complications of diabetes?**

Findings from the Diabetes Control and Complications Trial (DCCT) and the **United Kingdom Prospective Diabetes Study (UKPDS)** have clearly shown that aggressive and intensive control of elevated levels of blood sugar in patients with type 1 and type 2 diabetes decreases the complications of nephropathy, neuropathy, retinopathy, and may reduce the occurrence and severity of large blood vessel diseases. Aggressive control with intensive therapy means achieving fasting glucose levels between 70120 mg/dl; glucose levels of less than 160 mg/dl after meals; and a near normal hemoglobin A1c levels (see below). Studies in type 1 patients have shown that in intensively treated patients, diabetic eye disease decreased by 76%, kidney disease decreased by 54%, and nerve disease decreased by 60%. More recently the Epidemiology of Diabetes Interventions and **Complications.**

**The EDIC trial** has shown that type 1 diabetes is also associated with increased heart disease, like type 2 diabetes. However, the price for aggressive blood sugar control is two to three times increase in the incidence of abnormally low blood sugar levels (caused by the diabetes medications). For this reason, **tight control of diabetes to achieve glucose levels between 70 to120 mg/dl is not recommended for children under 13 years of age**, patients with severe recurrent hypoglycemia, patients unaware of their hypoglycemia, and patients with far advanced diabetes complications. To achieve optimal glucose control without an undue risk of abnormally lowering blood sugar levels, patients with type 1 diabetes must monitor their blood glucose at least four times a day and administer insulin at least three times per day. **In patients with type 2 diabetes, aggressive blood sugar control has similar beneficial effects on the eyes, kidneys, nerves and blood vessels.**

**What is the prognosis for a person with diabetes?**

**The prognosis of diabetes is related to the extent to which the condition is kept under control to prevent the development of the complications** (see preceding sections). Some of the more serious complications of diabetes such as kidney failure and cardiovascular disease, can be lifethreatening. Acute complications such as diabetic ketoacidosis can also be lifethreatening. Aggressive control of blood sugar levels can prevent or delay the onset of complications, and many people with diabetes lead long and full lives.

## SUMMARY

Choose More than 50 Ways to Prevent Type 2 Diabetes Reduce Portion **Sizes.**

**Use smaller portions sizes.** Portion size is the amount of food you eat, such as 1 cup of fruit or 6 ounces of meat. If you are trying to eat smaller portions, eat a half of a bagel instead of a whole bagel or have a smaller hamburger instead of a larger hamburger. Three ounces is about the size of your fist or a deck of cards.

**Put less on your plate**
- Drink a large glass of water 10 minutes before your meal so you feel less hungry.
- Keep meat, chicken, turkey, and fish portions to about 3 ounces.
- Share one dessert.

**Eat a smaller meal**
- Use teaspoons, salad forks, or childsize forks, spoons, and knives to help you take smaller bites and eat less.
- Make less food look like more by serving your meal on a salad on a breakfast plate.
- Eat slowly. It takes 20 minutes for your stomach to send a signal to your brain that you are full.
- Listen to music while you eat instead of watching TV (people tend to eat more while watching TV).
-

## A Holistic Approach to Understanding...

**Plate of food with proportions for each**

**How much should I eat?**
- Try filling your plate like this:
- 1/4 protein 1/4 grains
- 1/2 vegetables and fruit dairy (lowfat or skim milk)

**Move More Each Day**
- Find ways to be more active each day. Try to be active for at least 30 minutes, 5 days a week. Walking is a great way to get started and you can do it almost anywhere at any time. Bike riding, swimming, and dancing are also good ways to move more.
- If you are looking for a safe place to be active, contact your local parks department or health department to ask about walking maps, community centers, and nearby parks.

**Dance it away**
- Show your kids the dances you used to do when you were their age.
- Turn up the music and jam while doing household chores. Work out with a video that shows you how to get active.
- **Exercise that is aerobic (elevates your heart rate and breathing) for at least 30 minutes / day, 34 times per week, is essential to good diabetic and cardiovascular outcomes.**

### Let's go
- Deliver a message in person to a coworker instead of sending an email.
- Take the stairs to your office. Or take the stairs as far as you can, and then take the elevator the rest of the way.
- Catch up with friends during a walk instead of by phone.
- March in place while you watch TV.
- Choose a place to walk that is safe, such as your local mall.
- Get off of the bus one stop early and walk the rest of the way home or to work if it is safe. Better still, shed the car or bus and walk or cycle instead.

### Make Healthy Food Choices
**Find ways to make healthy food choices.** This can help you manage your weight and lower your chances of getting type 2 diabetes.

Choose to eat more vegetables, fruits, and whole grains. **Cut back on highfat foods like whole milk, cheeses, and fried foods.** This will help you reduce the amount of fat and calories you take in each day.

### Snack on a veggie
- Buy a mix of vegetables when you go food shopping.
- Choose veggie toppings like spinach, broccoli, and pep – pers for your pizza.
- Try eating foods from other countries. Many of these dishes have more vegetables, whole grains, and beans.

- Buy frozen and lowsalt (sodium) canned vegetables. They may cost less and keep longer than fresh ones.
- Serve your favorite vegetable and a salad with lowfat macaroni and cheese.

**Cook with care**
- Stir fry, broil, or bake with nonstick spray or lowsalt broth.
- Cook with less oil and butter. Avoid deep fried food.
- Try not to snack while cooking or cleaning the kitchen.
- Cook with smaller amounts of cured meats (smoked turkey and turkey bacon). They are high in salt.
- Cook with a mix of spices instead of salt.
- Try different recipes for baking or broiling meat, chicken, and fish.
- Choose foods with little or no added sugar to reduce calories.
- Choose brown rice instead of white rice.

**Eating healthy on the go**
- Have a big vegetable salad with lowcalorie salad dressing when eating out. Share your main dish with a friend or have the other half wrapped to go.
- Make healthy choices at fast food restaurants. Try grilled chicken (with skin removed) instead of a cheeseburger. Skip the fries and chips and choose a salad.
- Order a fruit salad instead of ice cream or cake. A colorful plate full of fruits and vegetables is hard to beat for health! (Mediterranean Diet)

### Rethink your drink
- Find a water bottle you really like (from a church or club event, favorite sports team, etc.) and drink water from it every day.
- Peel and eat an orange instead of drinking orange juice.
- If you drink whole milk, try changing to 2% milk. It has less fat than whole milk. Once you get used to 2% milk, try 1% or fatfree (skim) milk. This will help you reduce the amount of fat and calories you take in each day.

**Drink water instead of juice and regular soda.**

### Eat smart
- Make at least half of your grains whole grains, such as
- whole grain breads and cereals, brown rice, and quinoa.
- Use whole grain bread for toast and sandwiches.
- Keep a healthy snack with you, such as fresh fruit, a hand – ful of nuts, and whole grain crackers.
- Slow down at snack time. Eating a bag of lowfat popcorn takes longer than eating a candy bar.
- Share a bowl of fruit with family and friends.
- Eat a healthy snack or meal before shopping for food. Do not shop on an empty stomach.
- **Shop at your local farmers market for fresh, organic, non – GMO grown local food.**

### Keep track of how and what you eat
- **Make a list of food you need to buy before you go to the store.**

- **Keep a written record of what you eat for a week.** It can help you see when you tend to overeat or eat foods high in fat or calories.

## Read the label
- Compare food labels on packages.
- Choose foods lower in saturated fats, trans fats, cholesterol, calories, salt, and added sugars.

## Focus on the Food
Mindfulness has become as buzzworthy as cold pressed coffee. **One simple way to eat healthier may be to simply be mindful when eating.**

Mindful eating does not mean dieting or restrictions. It's more about taking a moment to take it in, truly enjoying and savoring what you eat. Food is more than nutrition; it is the sub – stance of life. There are a lot of methods out there, but we've simplified some of these for you.

Ponder: Before you eat, ask yourself, "**Am I really hungry? Or am I eating as a crutch for something else?**" Sometimes we think we are hungry when we're actually thirsty or bored or stressed. Do you need nourishment in the form of food, or do you need something else?

Appraise: When your food is in front of you, take a moment. How does it look? How does it smell? Do you really want it? Is it more than you need?

Slowly: Slow down, way down. Put your fork down between bites. Really chew your food and taste it. Slowing down helps your brain catch up with your stomach.

*Savor:* Really enjoy your food. How does the texture feel in your mouth? What are all the complex flavors you can taste? Take a moment to savor the satisfaction of each bite.

*Stop:* Stop when you're full. Sounds so obvious, right? By noticing when you are full and stopping, you may avoid unnecessary calories and indigestion.

### Take Care of Your Mind, Body, and Soul
Candles and oils

**You can exhale**
- Take time to change the way you eat and get active. 50. Try one new food or activity a week.
- Find ways to relax. Try deep breathing, taking a walk, or listening to your favorite music.
- Pamper yourself. Read a book, take a long bath, or meditate.
- Think before you eat. Try not to eat when you are bored, upset, or unhappy.

**Be Creative**

**Honor your health as your most precious gift.** There are many more ways to prevent or delay type 2 diabetes by making healthy food choices and moving more. Discover your own and share them with your family, friends, and neighbors.

**Diabetes booklet**

This booklet has charts to help you track the foods you eat and how much you move each day. There are many mobile

# A Holistic Approach to Understanding...

software applications and internetbased calculators that are also available for this purpose.

**Things to Remember**

- Talk to your doctor about your risk for getting type 2 diabetes and what you can do to lower your chances.
- **Take steps to prevent diabetes by making healthy food choices, staying at a healthy weight, and moving more every day.**
- Find ways to stay calm during your day. Being active and reading a good book can help you lower stress.
- Keep track of the many ways you are moving more and eating healthy by writing them down.
- Remember finally, setting the right eating and health care examples matter. The next generation develops its eating habits in large part from the previous general.

Katarzyna Dorosz

## HERBS

### Gymnema Sylvestre (Gurmar)

Gymnema Sylvestre is an incredible Ayurvedic herb that grows in tropical areas of India, Africa, and Australia. It has an ability to regulate the usage of glucose in body cells, and, as an effect, lower the bloodsugar level. It can also prevent the liver from producing excessive amounts of glucose and lower the level of cholesterol and triglycerides. Many people believe that Gymnema is one of the most effective herbs when it comes to diabetes treatment. Gymnema is a grapevine found in India. It has been used in Indian natural medicine since 600 BCE. It contains medicinal compounds that have the incredible ability to slow down the transportation of glucose from the digestive system to the blood. **Some doctors believe that Gymnema can help in the regeneration of beta cells that are producing insulin.** Let us look at the results of a study done in India on 22 patients with type 2 diabetes – every day, for 18 months patients consumed 400mg of Gymnema extract. It was found that this herb can significantly lower the glucose level in blood. What is more, tested patients were able to safely reduce the dose of their normal diabetes medications. 5 of them were able to maintain a stable bloodsugar without any other medications. This and many other studies had proven that **Gymnema has the ability to regulate the bloodsugar level by controlling the pancreatic production of insulin.**

## Cinnamon

Cinnamon can affect the bloodsugar level regulation and lipid profile of patients with type 2 diabetes. Cinnamon is loaded with powerful polyphenol antioxidants (also found in green tea and black tea). Consumption of cinnamon is useful in controlling the proper bloodsugar level, together with normally prescribed medications if needed.

## Cloves

According to clinical studies, cloves can strengthen the heart, liver, and eyes from the detrimental effects of diabetes. This spice contains 30 % antioxidants together with anthocyanins, and quercitrin. It has powerful antibacterial and antiseptic features. **Cloves have antiinflammatory and analgesic benefits**. Oil of cloves is used extensively as a topical anesthetic for tooth ache etc... It is an excellent dietary support for people with diabetes because of its beneficial metabolic effects. Other studies have established that eating 13 pieces of cloves daily for 30 days may significantly decrease the concentration of blood sugar and cholesterol.

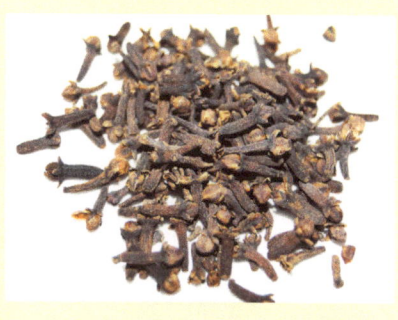

## Rosemary

This incredibly aromatic herb is commonly used as an addition to meat and soups. Rosemary can be also used as a natural medication, to sup – por t diabetes treatment.

Rosemary can assist in weight loss, which is especially important for people who have diabetes. Laboratory tests had proven that rosemary can significantly impact the levels of glucose, insulin, and lipids. After 4 weeks of supplying the rosemary extract, the bloodsugar level decreased by approximately 20%, chole – sterol 22%, triglycerides 24%.

## Oregano

Oregano is especially popular in Italian, Spanish and Medi – terranean cuisine. Many consider Oregano one of the most effective herbs, when it comes to diabetes management. Mexican scientists have established conclusively that oregano can reduce cellular oxidative stress by blocking the process of lipid peroxidation. Oregano can also prevent or at least slow down the effects of aging and kidneys damage. Why not add a bit of this aromatic and tasty herb to your food? Better still make up a mixture of your favorite herbs (Basil. Oregano, Rosemary etc...) as a mixture either fresh or dried to add to your cuisine. You can also mix oregano and/or basil with olive oil to make a salad dressing.

## Sage

The British Journal of Nutrition has studies that show that consumption of sage results in metabolic and endocrine effects remarkably similar to that of metformin. Remember to add it to your everyday meals. For ages, Sage has been used in traditional and natural medicine as a good way to lower the bloodsugar level.

One important warning: It is extremely important to remember, that consuming of sage together with diabetes medications can reduce the bloodsugar level too low excessively and cause symptoms of hypoglycemia (e.g. 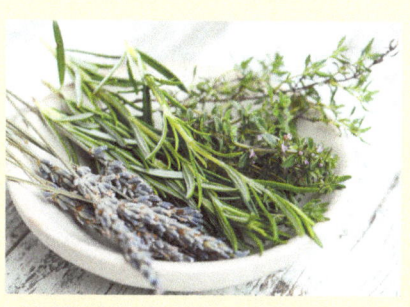 sweating, dizziness, shakiness etc…even drowsiness or loss of consciousness). **Ask your physician, before using herb remedies or supplements, and carefully follow your blood sugar level while using new herbs as adjunctive medical therapy.**

## Curry leaves

Curry leaves, or "kadi patta", are the leaves of the curry tree, scientifically known as Murraya koenigii Spreng. It belongs to the Rutaceae family. The plant is native to India and is usually found in tropical and subtropical regions. It is cultivated in various other countries including China, Australia,

Nigeria, and Ceylon. This spice that can help with regulating bloodsugar level by controlling the metabolism of carbohydrates. According to study results published in the International Journal of Development Research, Curry leaves are especially helpful and versatile in helping people with type 2 diabetes. This spice can lower bloodsugar in diabetics, both on an empty stomach and after meals. Curry leaf extract can also support the optimal functioning of the liver and kidneys. What is more, it can boost the formation of pancreatic cells, thereby boosting the production of insulin. The health benefits of curry leaves also include treating diarrhea, controlling diabetes, improving eyesight, and reducing stress. **Curry leaves contain various antioxidant molecules which aid digestion and correct an unhealthy good: bad cholesterol balance**. They are also believed to have cancerfighting properties.

## Garlic

Clinical studies have established that consumption of garlic can significantly reduce the level of glucose, cholesterol, triglycerides, urea, and many other toxic substances. Testing in rats, showed that **garlic can increase the amount of insulin**. Definitely, a good and tasty reason to add it to your diet. Garlic is extensively used in Mediterranean diets.

## Ginger

Ginger is well known for alleviating stomach ailments and supporting metabolism, which is especially important especially for people with diabetes, who are often struggling with many metabolismrelated issues. Ginger also can regulate the bloodsugar level.

## Turmeric

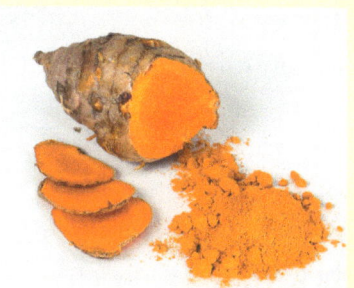

One of the most popular Indian spices, and one of the traditional ingredients of Indian curries. **Turmeric is well known all around the world- for its antibacterial, inflammatory, and antioxidant properties**. Turmeric has the ability to help the body maintain a stable blood – sugar level. For people with diabetes, that means better immunity also and less chances for acquiring infections. Turmeric can also lower glucose concentration and also ameliorate the lipid profile. With its antiinflammatory abilities, it can prevent joints problems, that often bother people with diabetes.

## Cayenne

**Cayenne pepper can stimulate the absorption of glucose by the intestines.** Results of studies published in 2006 in the European Journal of Pharmacology prove that adding this spice to food can help maintain optimal bloodsugar levels. Not only cayenne but also all the other kinds of pep

– pers share these antidiabetic and antiinflammatory properties. This is why they are so popular in traditional medicine not to mention their role in advancing the taste of many cuisines all around the world.

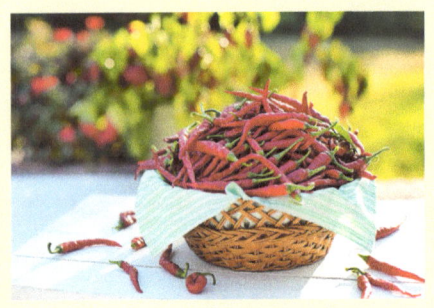

## Marjoram

Marjoram is not the most popular of all herbs, but it may help with diabetes treatment. It can reduce the production of **AGE – Advanced Glycation Endproducts**, that, according to the latest research, cause many sideeffects like damage to the eyes and arteries. Marjoram lowers the absorption of glucose and slows down the metabolism of absorbed carbo hydrates. Add it to your dinner every night– your meals will become more aromatic and you will help your body fight diabetes or even its tendency.

## Ginseng

Ginseng is a herb commonly used in the traditional Chinese medicine as one of the most effective bloodsugar control herbal supplements. Indian kind of that plant is incredibly advantageous for everybody, not only people with diabetes. Doctors all over the world are also testing the possibilities of its beneficial effects on memory and Alzheimer disease.

## EXERCISES

### Make it your routine

**Do you exercise enough?** Sadly, for most people probably not. It's a sad reality, especially for people with diabetes, that so many are sedentary when they could realize the benefits of being more active. Clinical studies worldwide have universally shown that only 39% of people with diabetes are exercising regularly. For many people without diabetes, the percentage is actually higher at 58%. A regular exercise workout is extremely important. Not only can it help to control the bloodsugar and better control the release of insulin, it beneficially improves cardiovascular health in innumerable ways. Exercising also helps to maintain the body's caloric balance and assists in weight loss.

It is important because so many patients with type 2 diabetes are overweight and have suffer the illeffects of morbid obesity. **Most physicians advocate regular physical activity as an important part of daily routine**. Easy, balanced training should be done at least 34 times a week for at least 30 minutes. It doesn't really have to be more complicated or intense.

### Walking

**Walking is simple easy and beneficial for all ages.** You do not need anything special to stay active by walking. The only thing you will need is a pair of comfortable shoes, that you most likely possess already. A quick energetic walk is a good cardio workout. The American Diabetes Associa tion recommends at least 3 cardio training sessions a week (~150 minutes). They also encourage against taking a break from exercising longer than 2 days. Walking should remain a regular lifelong habit.

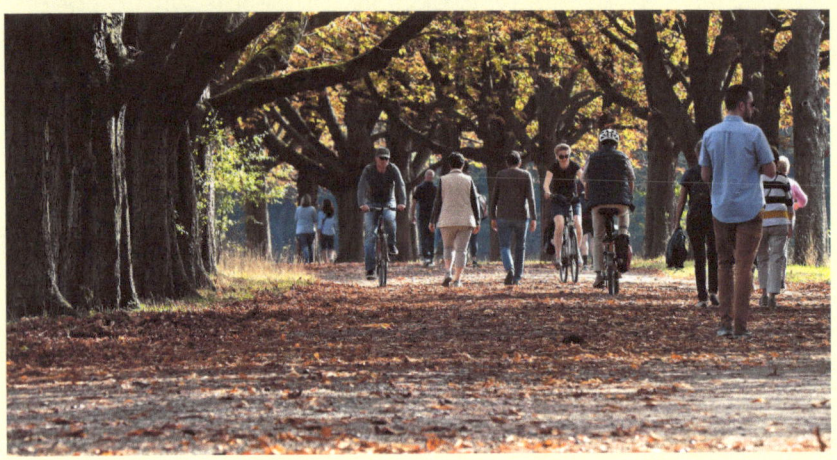

## Tai Chi

Tai Chi is a series of relaxing and balanced stylized movements (not an intense martial art) that has been a popular activity for ages in China. All evidence suggests that this kind of regular activity has a very positive effect for people with type 2 diabetes. **Tai Chi excels not only as a physical activity but also as an excellent relaxation technique**. It improves physical balance and musculoskeletal strength. Regular Tai Chi can not only offer a way to stay healthy and fit, but also to **slow down aging and reduce its effects**. You will need instruction on how to perform beneficial Tai Chi if you are a novice.

## Strength training

Strength training is also important as an adjunct to regular aerobic physical activity for people with diabetes. 23 strength training a week should be a part of the diabetes treatment routine. **It is important to remember to always take a break day between periods of training and never do it one day after another without pause – use "break" days to "mix in" other kinds of physical activity.** Every training session should combine 5 – 10 different exercises for different muscles groups. To have the best effect, one should do 34 sets of every exercise (1015 repetitions per set). Small dumb bells and ankle weights can assist in repetitive strength training.

## Yoga

Many have proven that yoga can bring many advantages for people with diabetes. It can help reduce adipose tissue, fight tissue insulin resistance, and even improve the functioning of nerves. All these effects are crucial for fighting the con – sequences of type 2 diabetes. As with Tai Chi, Yoga is great for relaxation and stress reduction. Stress can markedly increase, a patients' bloodsugar levels. That is why it's so important to remember effective relaxation techniques. Another advantage of Yoga is that you can do it as often as you want to – the more, the better. The Journal of Physical Activity and Health published in 2017 the results of studies showing that Yoga can even help fight depression. **Yoga is thus one of the very best activities to improve mood, improve glucose control, and accelerate weight loss for overweight diabetics.**

## Swimming

Swimming is great activity for people with type 2 diabetes and join problems because it is a relatively nonweight bearing exercise. One of the best specific advantages of this exercise is that it has no impact stress on the joints. Floating on the water brings no tension to your body or joints. It is also easier and, in some ways, less tiring than other activities, like jogging or walking. It also reduces the chance for foot scrapes and blisters that, for people with diabetes, are difficult to heal sometimes.

## Stationary Biking

Cycling offers an excellent cardiotraining activity that can strengthen your cardiovascular system, if not the whole body. Exercising on a stationary bike is a great activity for people with diabetes because the training can be done no matter what the outside weather conditions, and there is little risk of falls and injuries. It lessens the weight bearing stress compared with walling or running. **Cycling undoubtedly improves the blood circulation in the legs**. If you take up regular cycling, you can easily burn calories and maintain an ideal body weight.

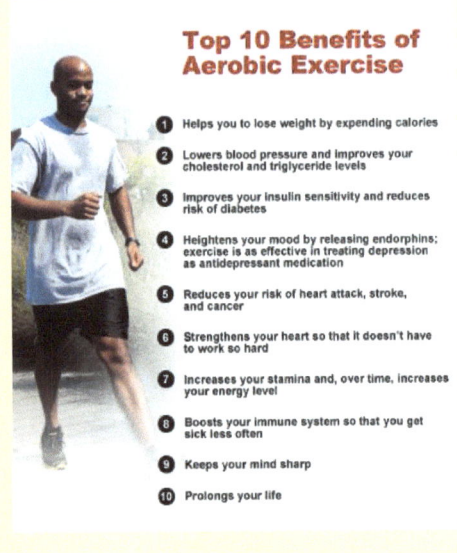

# Chapter 3
# Varicose veins

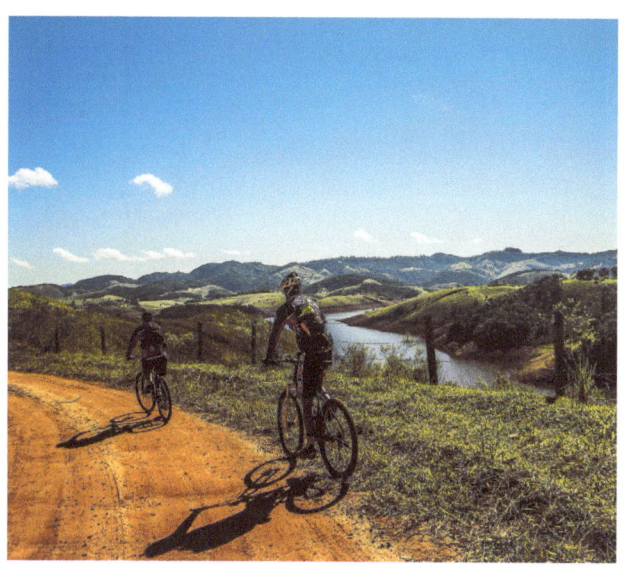

## What are varicose veins, why are they important, and how can we recognize them?

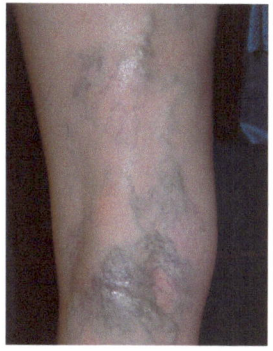
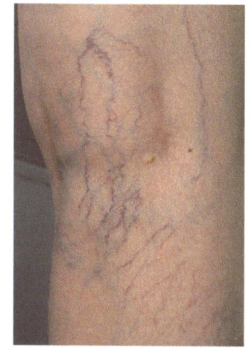
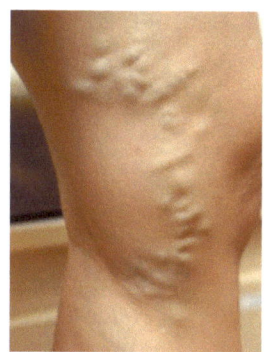

Types of varicose veins. Spider veins are pink or reddish – bluish and threadlike. Reticular veins are blue and stringlike. **True varicose veins are large rope or wormlike veins that bulge out from the skin surface.**

## What is venous disease and who is the most vulnerable to venous disease?

Veins return blood to the right side of the heart from all the body's organs and tissues. To reach the heart, the blood needs to flow upward against gravity from the leg veins. Calf muscles and the muscles in the feet need to contract with each step to squeeze the veins and force the blood upward. To keep the blood flowing up, and not back down, the veins contain oneway antigravity valves. **Chronic venous insufficiency (CVI)** occurs when these valves become damaged, allowing the blood to leak backward. Valve damage may occur as the result of aging, extended sitting or standing, or a combination of aging and reduced mobility. When the veins and valves are weakened to the point where it is difficult for the blood to flow upwards to the heart, the blood pressure in the veins stays elevated for long periods of time, leading to CVI. The distended varicose veins that result is often the first visible sign of this disease, also known as **chronic venous reflux disease.**

**CVI** commonly occurs as the result of a blood clot in the deep veins of the legs, a disease known as deep vein thrombosis (**DVT**). CVI also results from pelvic tumors and vascular malformations, and sometimes occurs for unknown reasons. Failure of the valves in leg veins to hold blood up against gravity leads to stagnation of blood within the veins, exudation of fluid and proteins into the tissues, resulting in swollen legs.

Chronic venous insufficiency that develops because of a prior DVT is also known as **postthrombotic syndrome**. As many as 30 percent of people with DVT will develop this problem within 10 years after diagnosis of a DVT.

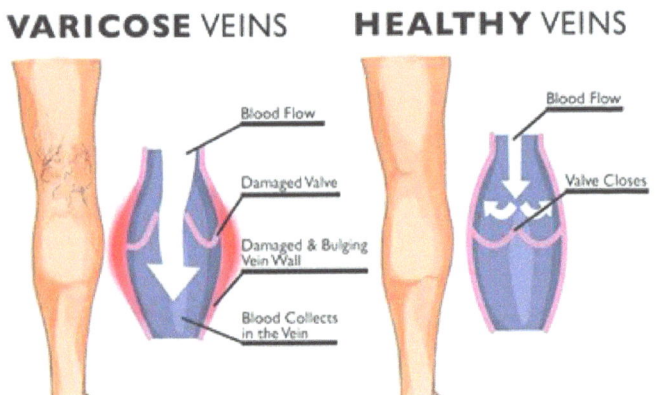

## What are the symptoms of chronic venous insufficiency?

The seriousness of CVI, along with the complexities of treatment, increase as the disease progresses. That is why it is so important to see your physician if you have any of the symptoms of CVI. The problem will not go away if you wait,

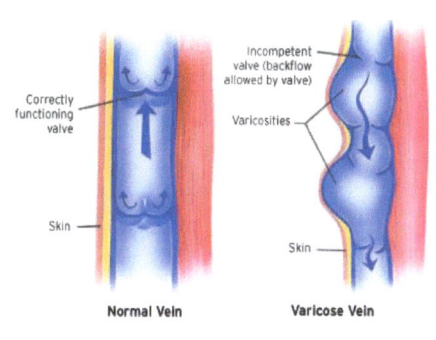

Normal Vein / Varicose Vein

and the earlier it is diagnosed and treated, the better your chances of preventing serious complications.

## Symptoms of varicose veins:
- Swelling in the lower legs and ankles, especially after extended periods of standing
- Aching or tiredness in the legs, especially after standing stationary for prolonged periods in one position
- New varicose veins
- Leatherylooking and/or pigmented skin on the legs around the ankles (the "gaiter" or sock zone above the ankle)
- Flaking or itching skin on the legs or feet
- Stasis ulcers (or "venous stasis" ulcers)

If CVI is not treated, the pressure and swelling increase until the tiniest blood vessels in the legs (capillaries) burst. When this happens, the overlying skin takes on a reddish-brown color and becomes extremely fragile and sensitive to being broken if bumped or scratched.

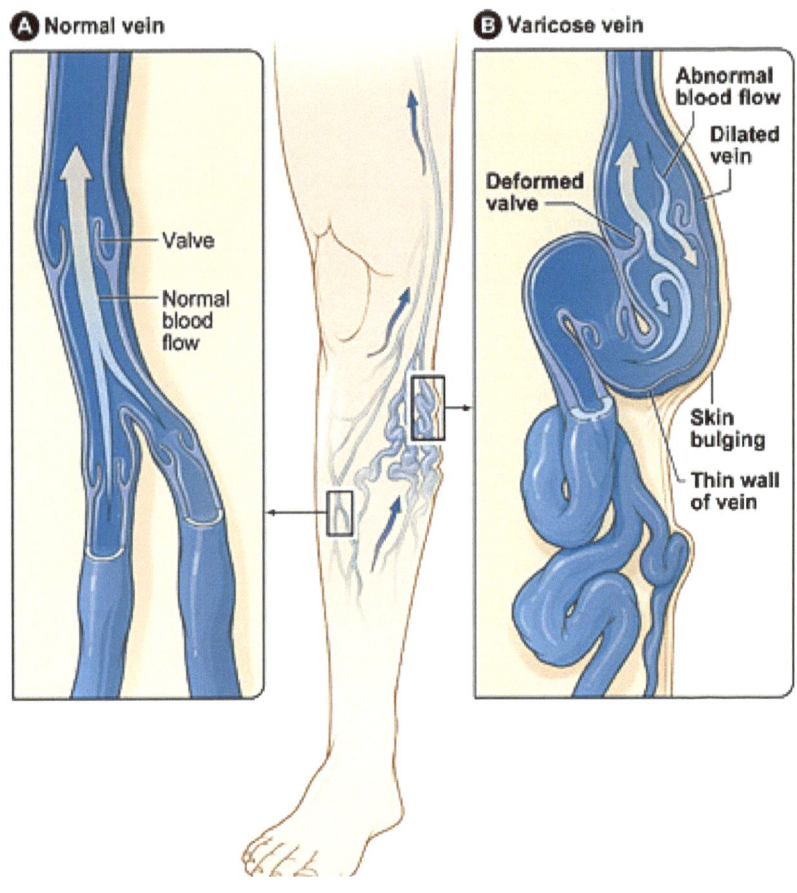

At the least, burst capillaries can cause local tissue inflammation, and also internal tissue damage. At worst, this leads to ulcers, open sores on the skin surface. These venous stasis ulcers can be difficult to heal and can become infected. When the infection is not controlled, it can spread to surrounding tissues, a condition known as cellulitis.

CVI is often associated with **varicose veins,** which are twisted, enlarged veins close to the surface of the skin. They can occur almost anywhere, but most commonly occur in the legs, but can occur on the arms, trunk, face, neck chest and abdomen even internally within the pelvis!

## What are the risk factors for chronic venous insufficiency?

If you have risk factors for CVI, you are more likely than other people to develop the disease. The most important risk factors are:

### Family History
Having close (first degree) family members who have varicose veins may raise your risk for the condition. About half of all people who have varicose veins have a CVI history in first degree. CVI or varicose vein reflux disease is one of the **most inheritable** cardiovascular conditions recognized.

### Older Age
Getting older may raise your risk for varicose veins. The normal wear and tear of aging may cause the valves in your veins to weaken and malfunction, leading to CVI.

### Gender
Women tend to get varicose veins more often than men. Hormonal changes that occur during puberty, pregnancy, and menopause (or with the use of birth control pills) may all raise

a woman's risk for varicose veins. Multiple pregnancies increase the risk for subsequent varicose vein disease development or accelerate preexistent CVI.

## Pregnancy

During pregnancy, the growing fetus puts pressure on the veins in the mother's legs. Varicose veins that occur during pregnancy usually get better within 3 to 12 months of delivery.

## Obesity

Being overweight or obese can put extra pressure on your veins. This can lead to development of varicose veins. For more information about overweight and obesity, go to the Health Topics on Overweight and Obesity.

## Lack of Movement

Standing or sitting for a long time, especially with your legs bent or crossed, may raise your risk for varicose veins. This is because staying vertical in one position for a long time may force your veins to work harder against gravity to pump blood to your heart.

## Leg Trauma

Previous blood clots or traumatic damage to the valves in your veins can weaken their ability to move blood upwards towards the heart, resulting in venous stagnation and increasing the risk for varicose veins.

## Who is affected by chronic venous insufficiency?

An estimated 40 percent of people in the United States have CVI. It occurs more frequently in people over age 50, and more often in women than in men.

## How is CVI diagnosed?

- **Clinical symptoms**
- **Visible skin changes and varicose veins**
- **Ultrasound and venous plethysmography (noninvasive venous function testing)**

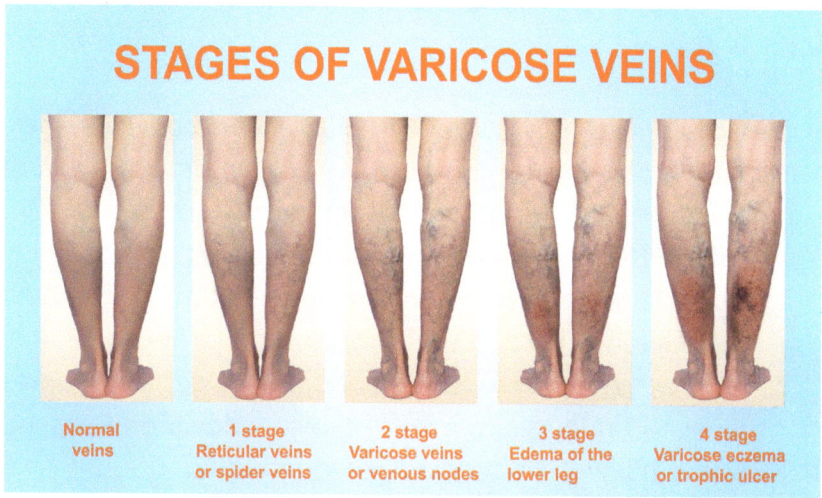

### Vascular Ultrasound

This is the "gold" standard in diagnosis of chronic venous reflux disease. To diagnose CVI, your doctor will perform a complete medical history and physical exam. During the physical exam, the doctor will carefully examine the circulation in your legs.

A test called a vascular or **duplex ultrasound** may be used to examine the blood circulation in your legs. During the vascular ultrasound, an ultrasound transducer (a small handheld device) is placed on the skin over the vein to be examined. The transducer emits ultrasound waves that bounce off the vein. These sound waves are recorded, and an image of the vessel is created and displayed on a monitor. **Vein valve leakage or insufficiency can be found and quantified using sophisticated venous doppler techniques.**

## How is chronic venous insufficiency treated or managed?

Like any disease, CVI is most treatable in its earliest stages. Vascular medicine or vascular surgery specialists typically recommend a combination of treatments for people with CVI. Some of the basic treatment strategies include:

- **Avoid long periods of standing or sitting:** If you must take a long trip and will be sitting for a long time, flex and extend your legs, feet, and ankles about 10 times every 30 minutes to keep the blood flowing in the leg veins. If you need to stand for long periods of time, take frequent breaks to sit down and elevate your feet.
- **Exercise regularly**. Walking is especially beneficial.
- **Lose weight i**f you are overweight. To check you body weight status online type BMI calculator in your browser or go the following link: https://www.cdc.gov/

healthyweight/assessing/bmi/adult_ bmi/english_bmi_calculator/bmi_calculator.html
- **Elevate your legs while sitting and lying down**, with your legs elevated above the level of your heart.
- Wear compression stockings while you are up and ambulated.
- The goals of treatment are to reduce the pooling of blood in the leg veins and prevent leg ulcers.

**Compression Stockings**

The most conservative approach is to wear properly fitting support hose (also called compression stockings). They come in different compression strengths varying from 8 to 10 mmHg, up to 40 to 50 mmHg. **You will need a prescription for any stockings with more than 20 mmHg compression.** These stockings should be **custom sized using specific circumferential ankle, calf and thigh measurements.**

**How can varicose veins be treated?**

Veins that are cosmetically unappealing or cause pain or other symptoms are prime candidates for treatment. There are two general treatment options: conservative measures, such as compression stockings or herbal remedies, and corrective measures such as sclerotherapy, surgery (vein ligation/stripping and excisional phlebectomy) , and a variety of vein ablation treatments (both thermal and glue or foam based vein ablation devices). Open surgical treatments requiring general anesthesia such as vein ligation and stripping are rarely used anymore. They have been replaced by more convenient safer office based vein ablation techniques that are just as efficacious and a lot less risky or painful.

## Conservative Treatments Compression Stockings

Graduated compression stockings are first line of defense and a mainstay of conservative management of venous disease. Graduated compression stockings create a tight pressure around the foot and ankle that gradually decreases as it moves up the leg. This "graduated compression" promotes the normal flow of blood up the leg. **Most vein specialist recommend that patients who suffer from spider veins, varicose veins, or venous insufficiency wear compression stockings**. Compression stockings can also be used to supplement other forms of treatment.

## Herbal Treatments

Natural plant medicines may strengthen the vein wall, reduce vein distension and leakiness, or decrease the inflammation that often accompanies vein reflux disease. **Horse chestnut extract** is the most commonly recommended herbal preparation for venous disease. Although there is no documented evidence of its efficacy, there are many anecdotal reports of beneficial effects on the symptoms of vein disease. **Bioactive flavonoids** extracted from citrus fruits e.g. Diosmin and Hesperidin, or a 9:1 combination of micronized purified flavonoid fraction (**MPFF**) e.g.

**Daflon**™, can all increase venous tone, improve lymphatic tissue drainage, and protect the tissue microcirculation. **MPFF can reduce lymphedema**, leg cramps, pelvic congestion symptoms, leg edema and rest – less leg symptoms.

## Sclerotherapy

Sclerotherapy is a common treatment for small (**spider veins**) and medium size (reticular) veins. A tiny needle is used to inject the veins with a solution (**sclerosant**) that chemically irritates and destroys the endothelium (lining) of the vein. In response, the veins collapse, scar and are reabsorbed. The surface veins are no longer prominently visible. Depending on the size and location of the veins, different types and strengths of sclerosants are used. With this procedure, veins can be dealt with at an early stage, helping to prevent further complications. A patient may need anywhere from one to several sclerotherapy sessions for any given vein region. Depending on the size, type, and number of veins being treated there may be need for one or several injections per session.

Sclerotherapy is usually performed in the doctor's office, and causes only minimal discomfort. **Generally, no "recovery" time is needed after sclerotherapy, and patients encouraged to resume their regular activities immediately.**

Dr. Sanjay Srivatsa

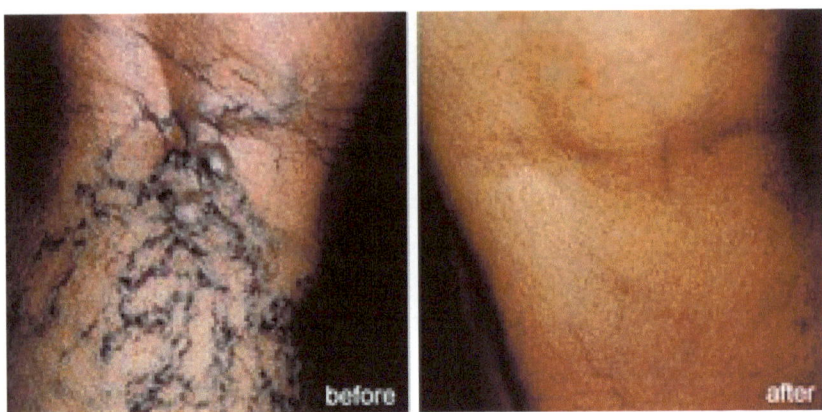

Varicose veins before and after sclerotherapy

Possible complications of sclerotherapy include inadvertent intraarterial injection, skin ulceration, hyperpigmentation (dark spots), telangiectatic matting (blush spots), superficial phlebitis, deep vein thrombosis (blood clots), and allergic reaction. Scarring, skin pigmentation, telangiectatic matting, and other complications are rare in skilled hands, but it is important to talk with your vein specialist about your options to understand the advantages and disadvantages of every treatment option.

**Endovenous Procedures**

There are essentially four types of endovenous procedures presently: Endovenous laser treatment, Endovenous radio frequency ablation, ultrasound guided sclerotherapy, and non-thermal, nontumescent based techniques e.g. Pharmacologic micro foam vein ablation (Varithena™) or mechanochemical vein ablation (Clarivein™).

**Clarivein**™ is a form of mechanically assisted sclerotherapy whereby a spinning blunt tipped needle is used to score the inner lining of the varicose vein and simultaneously sclerosant is infiltrated that then chemically destroys and scars the vein wall. It greatly enhances the efficacy of the sclerotherapy and enables its action in larger refluxing varicose veins.

## Endovenous Laser Treatment

Endovenous laser treatment is a minimally invasive, inoffice treatment alternative to surgical stripping of the great saphenous vein. Instead of removing the saphenous vein, it is sealed closed in place. The skin on the inside of the knee is anesthetized and a small laser fiber is inserted through a needle stick into the refluxing incompetent vein. Pulses of laser light are delivered inside the vein, which then cause heating of the the vein wall which then causes it to collapse, seal shut, and eventually regress into scar tissue over a period of several

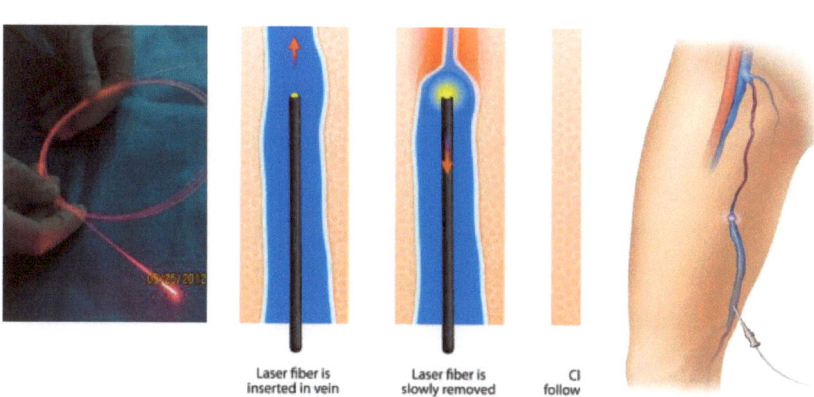

Laser fiber is inserted in vein

Laser fiber is slowly removed

Cl follow

weeks to months.

**This procedure is done inoffice under local anesthesia.** Following the procedure, a bandage or compression hose is placed on the treated leg. **Patients can walk immediately after the procedure** and most individuals are able to return to work the next day.

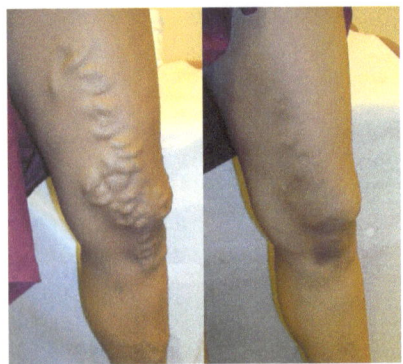

Before and after vein ablation photographs
**Endovenous Radio Frequency Ablation**

Endovenous Radio Frequency Ablation is a **minimally invasive, inoffice treatment alternative to surgical stripping of the great saphenous vein.** Instead of removing the saphenous vein, it is sealed closed in its place. The skin on the inside of the knee is anesthetized and a **radiofrequency catheter** is inserted into the damaged vein through a needle stick in the skin. The catheter delivers radiofrequency energy to the vein wall causing it to heat. As the vein is heated, it collapses, and seals shut, later to fibrose into scar tissue, as it heals over the next several weeks.

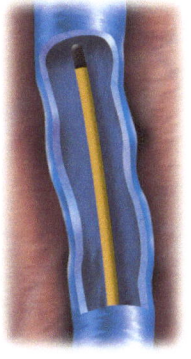 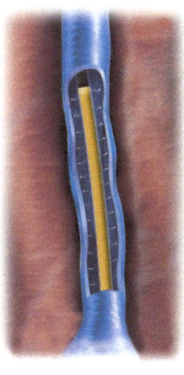 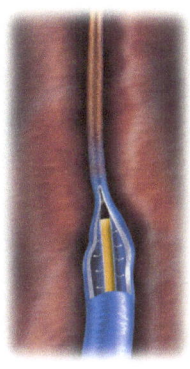

Disposable catheter inserted into vein | Vein heats and collapses | Catheter withdrawn, closing vein

**The procedure is generally done in an outpatient or inoffice setting, under local anesthesia.** Following the procedure, the catheter is removed, and a bandage or compression stocking is placed on the treated leg. Patients can walk immediately after the procedure and most individuals are able to return to work the next day or following day with use of compression stockings.

## NONTHERMAL TECHNIQUES

**ClariVein™ (Mechanically assisted chemical sclerotherapy)** ClariVein™ vein ablation uses a technique which is already commonly and successfully used to treat varicose veins, namely sclerotherapy. Sclerotherapy uses a sclerosing agent that dam – ages the inside of the vein causing scarring and closure of the target vein. Sclerotherapy works well on smaller varices but is not the optimal treatment for bigger veins like the saphenous veins. The ClariVein™ catheter solves these problems, by using a catheter with a rotating tip that disperses the sclerosant 360 degrees inside the varicose vein that is prescored by the rotating blunt tip needle, allowing successful treatment of larger veins. The physician gains access to the vein through a needle. Then the catheter is advanced to the top of the vein. Once in place the device is activated and pulled back slowly towards the feet. **This method does not use heat; therefore no tumescent anesthesia and needle sticks are necessary.** ClariVein™ is highly effective with comparable closure rates to thermal ablation. **No heat means no tumescent which means less needle injections** for anesthesia and greater patient.

## Ultrasound Guided Sclerotherapy

Ultrasound Guided Sclerotherapy is another inoffice treatment that has largely replaced surgical stripping. With sclerotherapy, the physician utilizes either a liquid or "foamed" sclerosant, while visually monitoring the filling and closure of the vein using ultrasound imaging. Ultrasound imaging is used to guide a needle into the abnormal vein and deliver sclerosant medication to destroy the lining of the blood vessel and seal it shut. **Ultrasound guided sclerotherapy is primarily used to treat medium to large sized veins beneath the surface of the skin.** Sclerotherapy can be used cosmetically to treat small reticular and spider veins in low chemical concentrations also.

A Holistic Approach to Understanding...

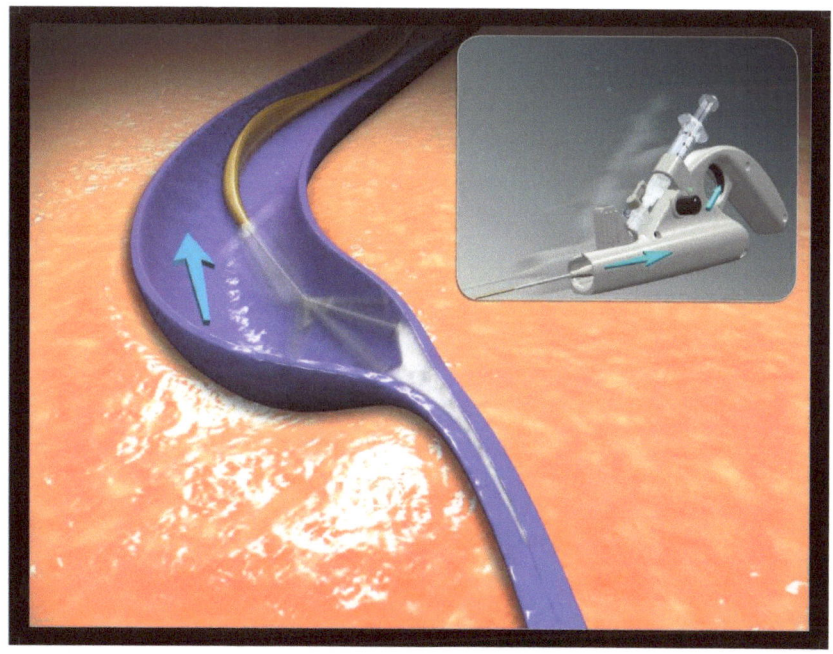

## Surgery

There are several surgical options including **vein ligation and vein stripping** available for the treatment of varicose veins. Surgery may be performed using local, spinal, or general anesthesia. Most patients return home the same day as the procedure. Surgery is generally used to treat large varicose veins. Hospital based vein stripping and ligation surgeries requiring general anesthesia and nowadays play a minor and diminishing role in the treatment of CVI and varicose vein disease, which best done under local anesthesia in the office setting, making it safer, less painful and more expeditious for

the patient.
## Traditional Surgical Ligation & Stripping

Traditional ligation and stripping of the great saphenous vein is usually performed in a hospital operating room or outpatient surgical center under general anesthesia. An incision is made in the groin, and the saphenous vein is tied off at its origin. Then a series of incisions are made in the leg and a wire "stripper" is inserted into the abnormal veins, which are then stripped out. Possible complications of vein stripping are damage to surrounding nerves resulting in numbness, damage to lymphatic tissue leading to lymphedema and chronic leg swelling. The surgery also leaves incision scars; however, this treatment can provide relief to patients suffering from serious venous disorders. **The role of vein ligation, stripping and excisional phlebectomy under general anesthesia has regressed in favor of endovascular office based minimally invasive vein ablation techniques performed in the office under local anesthesia.**

## Ambulatory Phlebectomy

Ambulatory phlebectomy is a method of surgical removal of surface varicose veins. Ambulatory phlebectomy is usually performed in a doctor's office using local anesthesia.

The area surrounding the varicose vein clusters is flooded with anesthetic fluid. A needle is then used to make a puncture next to the varicose vein and a small hook is inserted through the needle hole and the varicose vein is grasped and removed from the body. The punctures typically leave small or nearly imperceptible scars. After the vein has been removed by phlebectomy, a bandage and/or compression stocking is worn for a short period. **Ambulatory phlebectomy** is often performed in conjunction with minimally invasive endovenous catheter procedures. Possible complications of ambulatory phlebectomy are allergic reaction to the local

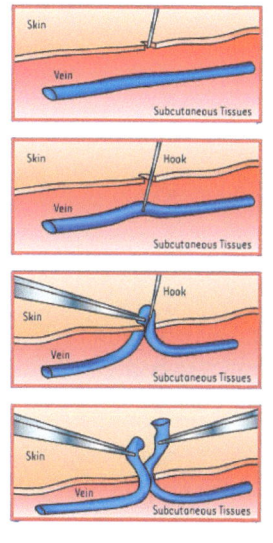
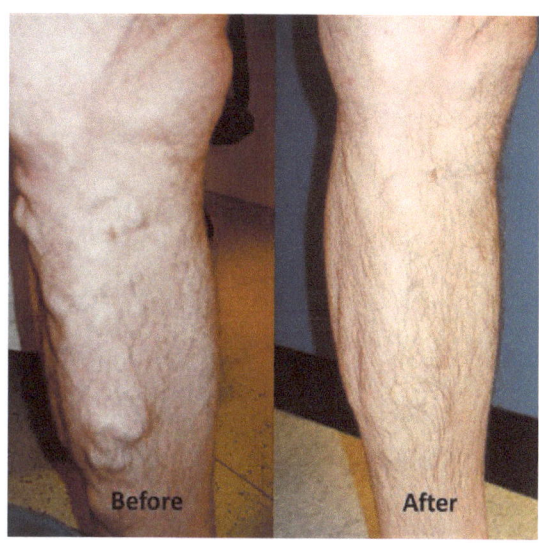

anesthetic and local numbness.

Varicose veins before and after ambulatory phlebectomy

## LightBased Treatments

**Laser and intense pulsed light (IPL)** can be used externally on the skin to treat small spider veins and facial redness. A light beam is pulsed through the skin and into the veins in order to seal them off and cause them to shrink and scar. Lightbased treatment is generally used only to treat small veins. Treatments may be combined with sclerotherapy, and multiple treatments are usually required.

**How can varicose veins be avoided?**

To reduce your risk of developing varicose veins and CVI, follow these guidelines:
- Eat a healthy balanced diet
- Quit smoking
- Exercise regularly
- Avoid wearing restrictive clothing such as tight girdles/belts
- Lose weight if you are overweight

If you have CVI and venous reflux symptoms and signs, **use compression stockings whenever up and ambulated for prolonged periods**, especially if you have CVI and venous reflux symptoms and signs.

## A few important rules to follow for varicose vein management

### Regular exercise

Regular exercise can improve the blood circulation into and out of the legs. It also helps to lower the resting venous blood pressure in the leg veins, which is also an important factor for those experiencing venous circulatory problems. Pick an activity that is challenging enough to elicit beneficial effects but, not so intense to be prohibitive. Good options to consider here may be swimming, walking, cycling or yoga.

### Compression stockings

You can easily buy these in any good medical equipment store. **Stockings work by placing compressive force externally to support the vein walls thereby reducing vein reflux and supporting muscle function**.

Properly fitted stockings can really improve the blood circulation by improving the efficiency of the veins in transporting the blood to the heart. The benefits of wearing compression stocking are noticeable for patients even after the first week of using them and persist indefinitely thereafter. Patients describe almost instantaneously feeling less pain caused by the varicose veins after wearing stockings. **Compression stockings should never be bought "off the shelf" but always based on recent accurate custom measurements of**

**the thigh, calf and ankles.** Only then can the appropriate compression pressure for treatment be obtained.

**Essential oils**

Clinical studies have shown consistently that horse chestnut extracts/essential oil can help to ease the pain, itching, and sensation of heaviness of varicose veins and lower leg vein disease. Physicians have used pinecone seed essential oils to reduce the swelling that is also one of the common effects of varicose veins and CVI. The horse chestnut tree (**Aesculus hippocastanum**) produces a seed that is used as a dietary supplement extract. **Horse chestnut seed extract (HCSE)** is a rich source of a nutrient called aescin which is believed to be the biologically active compound. Horse chestnut extract works in multiple ways to support the health of your capillaries and veins. HCSE is a direct venotonic substance for veins and valves, and a source of nourishment that enhances their structural strength. It has been shown to close small endothelial gaps in the vein wall lining that allow fluid leakage.

In addition to its structural support for veins and valves HCSE has a regulating function relating to both capillaries and veins. Its actions are unique and fascinating. Horse chestnut seed extract (HCSE) relaxes the endothelial lining of vessels, by enhancing beneficial nitric oxide release, while also reducing inflammation. This helps maintain a healthy blood pressure. **HCSE helps reduce capillary leakage of excess extracellular fluid into the tissues**. By supporting the structural integrity of veins and valves, HCSE improves the pumping efficiency of the veins against gravity. HCSE helps improves flow through the closely related tissue drainage **lymphatic system** of the legs – another pressure system that can get backed up and cause circulation problems. This is a unique combination of beneficial HCSE actions that markedly improve the venous circulation of the legs.

## How to use essential oils?

Always, dilute down any essential oils with a base carrier oil (e.g. coconut or avocado oil) or alternatively in aloe vera gel or unscented body lotion and use them topically via an aromatherapy diffuser.

### Change your diet

Keep in mind a few important facts about your diet. Diets rich with high potassium content can counter hyper – tension and water retention in the body. What are these products? The best source of potassium is almonds, pistachios, lentils, white beans, potatoes, leafy vegetables, salmon, and tuna. On the other hand, salty products (large sodium content) are water retaining in their effects. Food high in soluble fiber can blunt the sugar and insulin spike after meals that have been linked to adverse metabolic effects and cardiovascular disease. **These fibrous foods are able to blunt the glucose rise in the blood as well as help to prevent constipation**. Foods with high fiber content are nuts, seeds, legumes, grains. Remember that whole grain products are always preferable.

## Consume more flavonoids

Food with high flavonoids content have a salutary effect as a varicose vein treatment. They improve the blood circulation, promotes the lowering of arterial blood pressure, and relaxes the vasculature. All these features are important for preventing and treating varicose veins and venous insufficiency. Food products that contain a lot of flavonoids include onions, bell peppers, spinach, broccoli, citrus fruits, grapes, apples, berries, cocoa, and garlic.

## Herbal remedies

According to the National Institute of Health (NIH), consuming grape seeds (Vitis vinifera) may decrease the swelling of legs and other varicose veins symptoms. Some prescription medications may negatively interact with grape seeds, so it is always better to ask a physician before using any herbal remedies, especially if you regularly take multiple medications.

## Keep your legs elevated when seated

Raising your legs and keeping them above, or at the same height as the heart may have a helpful effect on your blood circulation and varicose vein symptoms. This maneuver lowers the hydrostatic blood pressure in the leg veins and uses the effect of gravity to improve the return of blood from the extremities back to the heart. Bear in mind, that especially during and after long periods of sitting or standing in one position, people with varicose veins are greatly benefited by **wearing compression stockings during upright activity** and by leg elevation and / or massage to clear dependent fluid at the end of a day. It is better to wear the compression stockings starting as soon as possible in the morning and retain them until the evening.

**Massage**

Gentle massage of your legs may improve the blood circulation and lessen the pain from venous stagnation. You can use essential oils to intensify the effect. Remember, firm compression is not actually necessary.

**Keep moving**

Avoid sitting for long periods of time. If you have to, take little breaks, change your position, do some mobilization exercises. Staying in a sitting position for prolonged time periods is not beneficial. If you are sitting, try to avoid crossing your legs. Keep them parallel on the floor to maintain the optimal blood circulation.

## HERBS:

### Chestnut seeds

These contain a lot of saponins – like aescin, which relax and support blood vessels, heal venous inflammations, and prevent the destruction of hyaluronic acid – thereby slowing down the aging of the circulatory system.

### Chestnut flowers

They contain not only aescin but also other bioactive flavonoids that have all the protective features for varicose veins. Flavonoids are crucial for the physiologic functioning of blood vessels – lack of these may promote vascular aging and allow vascular damage to accelerate.

### Berries

Especially **chokecherry, blueberries, and elderberry**. These are a good source of easy absorbable flavonoids. Making these a good substantial proportion of your diet to promote strong and healthy blood vessels.

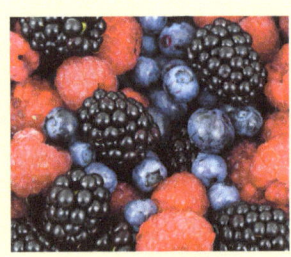

### Rue (Rutaceae, citrus family)

This is a good source of kind of flavonoids called **Rutin** – one of the most popular flavonoids, an ingredient of many venous medications. Allnatural substances extracted from such herbs can be more effective than artificial ones and are often used in medicinal products. Nature knows best! Rutin (quercetin/rutoside) is a bioflavonoid found in buck wheat, Eucalyptus, Japanese pagoda tree, figs, apples, and green tea that prevents oxidative damage to vessel walls and lowers BP/cholesterol. It strengthens capillaries, maintains flexibility and neutralizes free radicals generated by inflammation.

**Buckwheat herb**

This herb is the best collected in early Spring. It contains 5% Rutin.

**Sea buckthorn**

Excellent source of vitamin C that is crucial for the right absorption of flavonoids. Vitamin C also has antiinflammatory features and can ameliorate leg swelling.

**Gingko**

Gingko leaves improve the blood circulation, have antiinflammation properties, and help to eliminate swelling of the tissues. Gingko also contains antioxidants that slow down the biological aging of blood vessels.

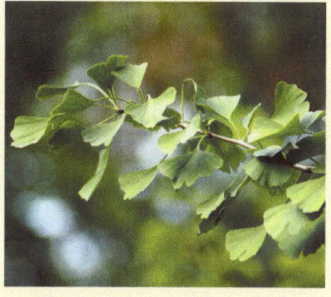

## Arnica flowers

Arnica contains large amounts of **sesquiterpenes** that are easily absorbed by tissues. They have the ability to reduce swelling and inflammation – problems fairly frequent in people with varicose veins.

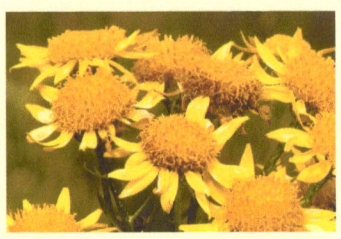

**Threelobe beggarticks** (Bidens tripartite) – one of my favorite herbs. It contains 14 different kinds of flavonoids! It also has antiinflammatory and antioxidant features. An essential oil of that herb is perfect for all kinds of skin irritation, swelling and itching.

**Pennywort** – this herb is famous for its features used in preventing and treating of varicose veins. It can activate the synthesis of collagen. Strong collagen scaffolds are crucial for blood vessels strength and functioning.

## Effective varicose veins treatment should be a composition of 3 elements.
- Renewing, strengthening, and improving the flexibility of blood vessels.
- Reducing the swelling and inflammation around blood vessels.
- Improving blood circulation and lowering blood pressure in the brain – lowering the chance of stroke.

## Using herbs as a part of varicose veins treatment has many positive benefits:

- Blood vessels become stronger and more resistant.
- Stabilization of the blood pressure.
- Weight loss promotes reduction in intraabdominal pressure thereby decreasing the hydrostatic pressure in the leg veins.
- Improving blood circulation in the brain – lowering the chance of stroke.
- Reducing the problems of hemorrhoids.
- Improving immunity – rendering your body less vulnerable to infections.
- Cosmetics that contain these types of herbs also have great antiaging features for your skin.

## EXERCISING – 12 RULES

### Talk to your doctor

Before starting a new kind of physical activity make sure, that it's safe and good for your particular situation.

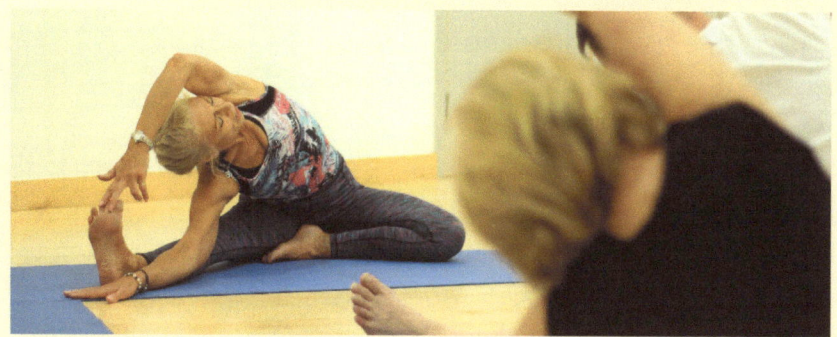

## Listen to your body

Always follow the "voice" of your body. Carefully observe and do not ignore any signals. If you feel any pain, or you feel like that any kind of activity is making your symptoms worse, stop it and consult with your doctor.

## Always do preexercise stretching to warmup

Start every activity with a warmup period. This prepares your body for the action to come and prevents muscle injuries.

## Walk as much as you can

Walking is the easiest exercise that you can do. When the weather allows, take a stroll outside and enjoy the nature or neighborhood. On inclement days, you can always go to the mall or use the treadmill or a stationary bike. While walking, the blood circulation is stimulated by the leg muscle contraction.

## Ride a bike

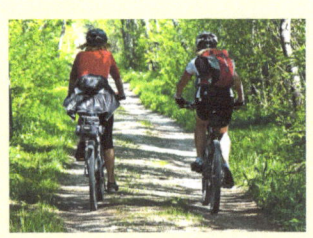

Go and take a ride on a bike or use a stationary one. Cycling uses all the leg muscles, and this obviously improves the blood circulation.

## Swim

Swimming has many advantages, not only for people with varicose veins. Swimming supports the blood circulation through the legs while maintaining the legs at the same level as the heart. It is considered one of the best aerobic non-weight bearing exercises available.

### Work out your thighs

The muscles of your thighs help to propel the blood upwards from your legs. An easy, but effective exercise is sitting down in a chair and standing up – without the aid of the arms. Repeat this 1015 times, take a break and repeat another 2 series.

### Cool down and stretch

After every training session, remember the importance of a "cool down" period. Slow down, breath with your nose, and do some light stretching. This is important to prevent muscle injury.

### Do not hold your breath

Always remember the importance of correct breathing, no matter how intense the exercise is. Holding the breath impedes the return of blood from the lower extremities and does little to correct the oxygen deficits that build up during exercise.

### Do not try to lift large weights

This type of heavy weightlifting increases the hydrostatic pressure in the lower body. If you really want to do some weightlifting, consult with your doctor and together set appropriate limits.

**Physical activity is very important, but everyone should remember to maintain a healthy and balanced diet.**

# Chapter 4
# Cholesterol

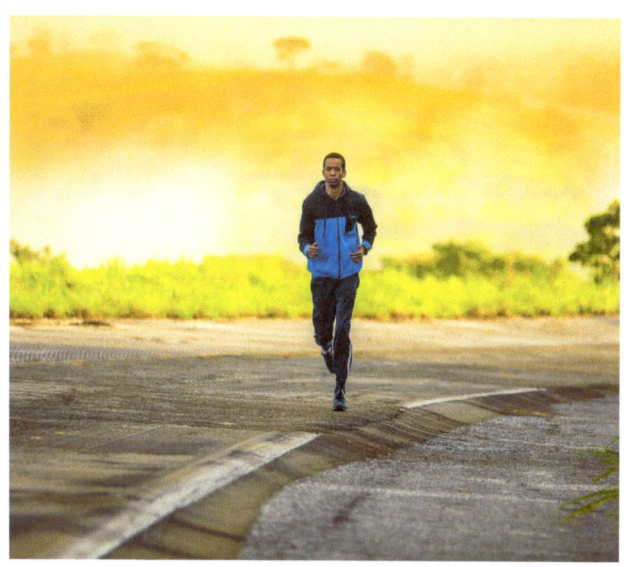

## LOWERING ELEVATED CHOLESTEROL: WHY?

### What is cholesterol?

Cholesterol is a chemical compound that the body requires for use as a building block for cell membranes and for hormones like estrogen and testosterone. The liver produces about 80% of the body's cholesterol and the rest comes from dietary sources like meat, poultry, eggs, fish, and dairy products.

Foods derived from plants contain no cholesterol. Cholesterol content in the bloodstream is regulated by the liver. After a meal, cholesterol in the diet is absorbed from the small intestine then metabolized and stored in the liver. As the body requires cholesterol, the liver secrets it. When too much cholesterol is present in the body, it can build up in deposits called plaque within the walls of arteries, causing them to narrow.

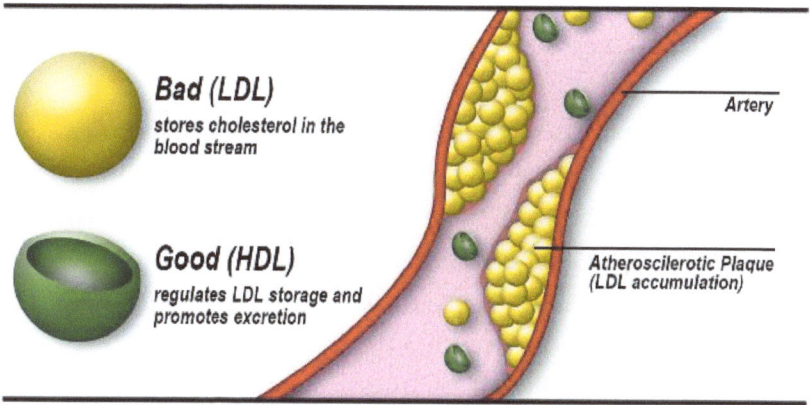

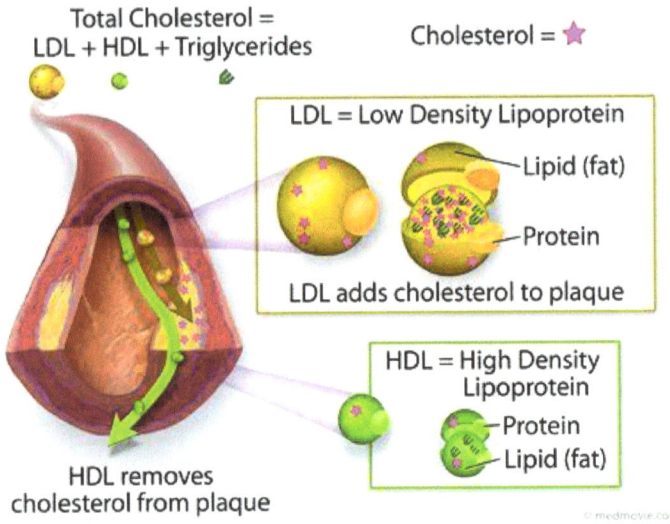

**Examples of foods high in cholesterol:**

- Egg yolks
- Shellfish like shrimp
- Processed meats like bacon
- Baked goods such as pies and cakes sometimes made with animal fats like lard and butter

**What are the different types of cholesterol?**

Cholesterol does not travel freely through the bloodstream. Instead, it is attached or carried by **lipoproteins** (lipo = fat) in the blood. There are three types of lipoproteins that are categorized based upon how much protein there is incorporated in relation to the amount of cholesterol.

| Healthy Blood Cholesterol Levels, by Age and Sex | | | | |
|---|---|---|---|---|
| Demographic | Total Cholesterol | Non-HDL | LDL | HDL |
| Age 19 or younger | Less than 170 mg/dL | Less than 120 mg/dL | Less than 100 mg/dL | More than 45 mg/dL |
| Men age 20 or older | 125 to 200 mg/dL | Less than 130 mg/dL | Less than 100 mg/dL | 40 mg/dL or higher |
| Women age 20 or older | 125 to 200 mg/dL | Less than 130 mg/dL | Less than 100 mg/dL | 50 mg/dL or higher |

**Lowdensity lipoproteins (LDL)** contain a higher ratio of cholesterol to protein and are thought of as the **"bad" cholesterol.** Elevated levels of LDL lipoprotein increase the risk of heart disease, stroke, and peripheral artery disease, by helping form cholesterol plaque along the inside of artery walls. Over time, as plaque buildup (plaque deposits) increases, the artery narrows (**atherosclerosis**) and blood flow decreases. If the plaque ruptures, it can cause a blood clot to form that prevents further blood flow. This clot is the root cause of a heart attack or myocardial infarction, when the clot occurs in one of the coronary arteries in the heart.

**Highdensity lipoproteins (HDL)** are made up of a higher level of protein and a lower level of cholesterol. These tend to be thought of as "good" cholesterol. The higher the HDL to LDL ratio, the better it is for the individual because such ratios can potentially be protective against heart disease, stroke, and peripheral artery disease.

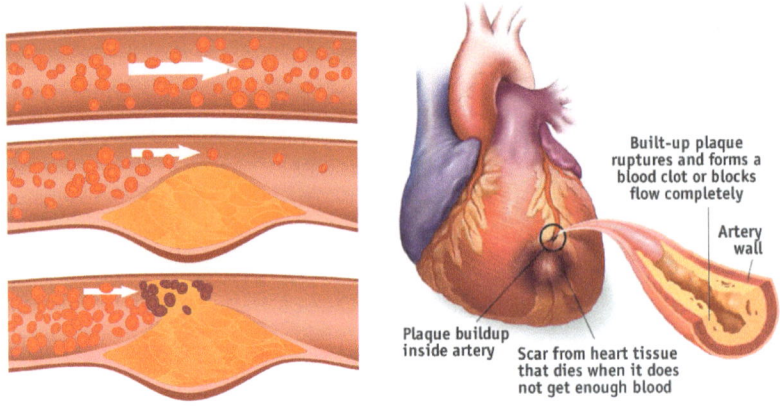

**Very lowdensity lipoproteins (VLDL)** contain even less protein than LDL. VLDL like LDL has been associated with plaque deposits.

Triglycerides (a type of fat) may increase cholesterol containing plaques if levels of LDL are high and HDL are low. Total cholesterol score is the sum of HDL cholesterol, LDL cholesterol and ~20% of triglycerides as determined by a blood test. A high adverse lipid score indicates an increased risk for developing cardiovascular disease and/or strokes.

Many online internet or mobile application based atherosclerotic risk calculators are available from reliable sources e.g. American College of Cardiology. One example is the 10 year ASCVD risk calculator which is accessible at

**http://tools.acc.org/ASCVDRiskEstimatorPlus/#!/calculate/estimate/**

## What are LDL and HDL Cholesterol?

LDL cholesterol is called **"bad" cholesterol,** because elevated levels of LDL cholesterol are associated with an increased risk of coronary heart disease, stroke, and peripheral arterial disease. LDL lipoprotein deposits cholesterol along the inside of artery walls, causing the formation of a hard, thick substance called cholesterol plaque.

| National Cholesterol Education Program Cholesterol Guidelines | | | |
|---|---|---|---|
| | Desirable | Borderline High | High |
| Total Cholesterol | Less than 200 | 200 - 239 | 240 and higher |
| LDL Cholesterol (the "bad" cholesterol) | Less than 130 | 130 - 159 | 160 and higher |
| HDL Cholesterol (the "good" cholesterol) | 50 and higher | 40 - 49 | Less than 40 |
| Triglycerides | Less than 200 | 200 - 399 | 400 and higher |

**HDL cholesterol** is called the **"good cholesterol"** because HDL cholesterol particles prevent atherosclerosis by extracting cholesterol from the artery walls and metabolizing them via the liver. Thus, high levels of LDL cholesterol and low levels of HDL cholesterol (high LDL/HDL ratios) are risk factors for atherosclerosis, while low levels of LDL cholesterol and high levels of HDL cholesterol (low LDL/HDL ratios) are desirable and protect against heart disease and stroke.

1 mmol/l = 38.66976 mg/dl or 1 mg/dl = 0.02586 mmol/l
To convert cholesterol levels from milligram per deciliter, mg/dl to millimole per liter, mmol/L multiply the mg/dl result by 0.02586 mmol/l or use the online calculator at
**http://www.onlineconversion.com**

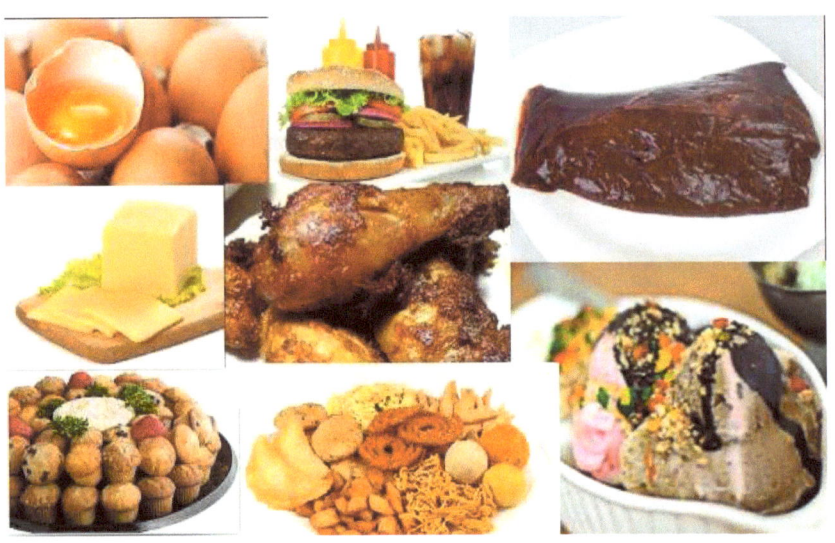

**Why is high cholesterol dangerous?**

Elevated cholesterol levels are just one of the key risk fac – tors for heart disease, stroke, and peripheral artery disease. The mechanism involving cholesterol in all three diseases is the same; plaque buildup within arteries decreases blood flow affecting the function of the cells and organs that these blood vessels supply.

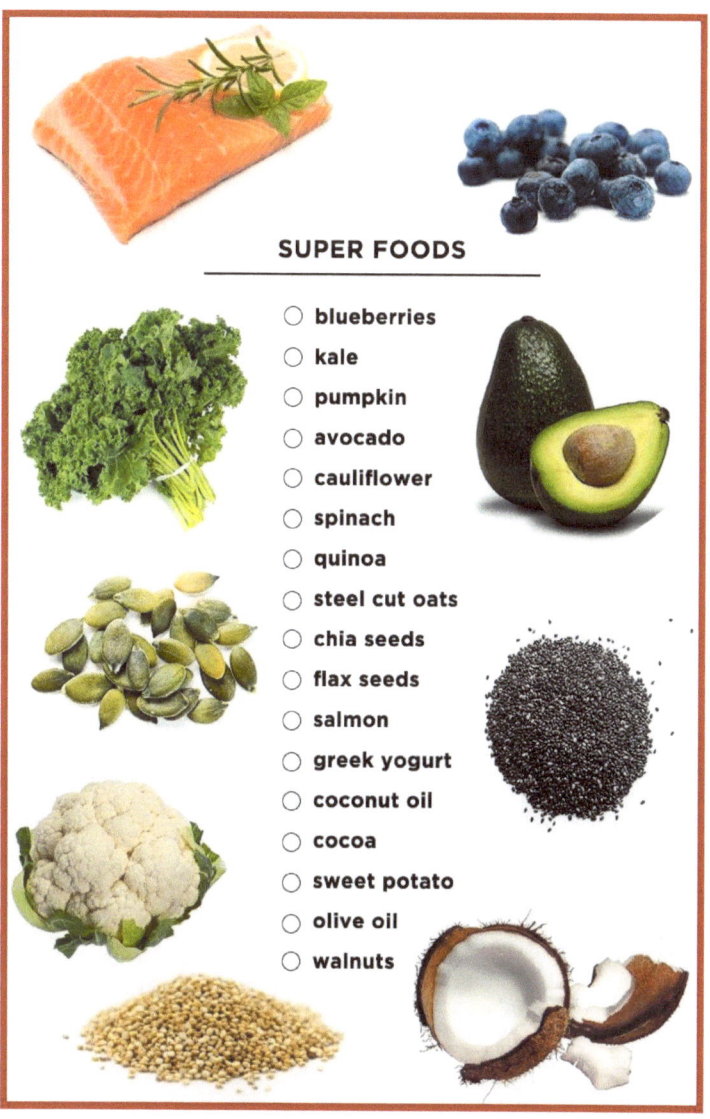

**SUPER FOODS**

- blueberries
- kale
- pumpkin
- avocado
- cauliflower
- spinach
- quinoa
- steel cut oats
- chia seeds
- flax seeds
- salmon
- greek yogurt
- coconut oil
- cocoa
- sweet potato
- olive oil
- walnuts

**Atherosclerotic heart disease** or narrowed coronary arteries in the heart can cause the symptoms of angina when the heart muscle is not provided with enough oxygen to function. Decreased blood supply to the brain may be due to narrowed small arteries in the brain or because the larger carotid arteries in the neck may become blocked. This can result in a **transient ischemic attack (TIA)** or stroke.

**Peripheral artery disease** describes gradual atherosclerotic plaque narrowing of the arteries that supply blood to the legs. During exercise, if the legs do not get enough blood supply, they can develop pain, called **claudication**. Other arteries in the body may also be affected by plaque buildup causing them to narrow, including the mesenteric arteries (intestines) and the renal arteries (kidneys).

**Where does cholesterol come from?**

The liver is responsible for managing the levels of LDL in the body. It manufactures and secretes LDL into the bloodstream. There are receptors on liver cells that can "monitor" and adjust the LDL levels. However, if there are fewer liver cells or if they do not function effectively, the LDL level may rise. Diet and genetics both play a factor in determining a person's cholesterol levels. There may be a genetic predisposition for **familial hypercholesterolemia** (hyper=more = cholesterol + emia=blood) where the number of liver receptor cells is low and LDL levels rise causing the potential for atherosclerotic heart disease at a younger age. In the diet, cholesterol comes from saturated fats that are found in meats, eggs, and dairy products. Excess saturated fat intake can cause LDL levels in the blood to rise. Some vegetable oils made from coconut, palm, and cocoa are also high in saturated fats.

## Lowering Your Cholesterol Levels

**What are normal cholesterol levels?**

Blood tests are required to measure total cholesterol and lipoproteins. For a complete lipoprotein analysis, the patient should be fasting for at least 12 hours.

### Cholesterol Risk Guidelines

Total Cholesterol (mg/dL)

| | |
|---|---|
| < 200 | Desirable |
| 200 to 239 | Borderline high |
| > 240 | High |

**HDL cholesterol (mg/dL)**

| | |
|---|---|
| < 40 | Low |
| > 60 | High |

**LDL cholesterol (mg/dL)**

| | |
|---|---|
| < 100 | Optimal |
| 100 to 129 | Near Optimal |
| 130 to 159 | Borderline high |
| 160 to 189 | Near high |
| > 190 | High |

**The goal is to have patients modify lifestyle and diet to maintain cholesterol levels within the normal range.** It is important to remember that HDL may protect a patient from heart disease, and it may occasionally be a treatment goal to raise an excessively low level of HDL. It remains an unfulfilled goal of lipid therapy to find a safe, effective way to raise HDL levels and thereby improve cardiovascular outcomes. Low HDL levels are associated with high triglycerides levels. By treating high TG's, the HDL level rises automatically.

**Which foods can help lower cholesterol?**

Diet guidelines can help to lower cholesterol levels. It may be a challenge to read the nutritional contents on food packaging and on restaurant menus or to do the math, but the benefit will decrease the risk of heart attack and stroke.

- **Limit total fat intake to less than 25% to 35% of your total calories each day.**
- **Limit saturated fat intake to less than 7% of total daily calories.**
- **Limit transfat intake to less than 1% of total daily calories.**

## LOWER IS BETTER WHEN IT COMES TO LDL CHOLESTEROL AND TRIGLYCERIDES

The remaining fat should come from sources of monounsaturated and polyunsaturated fats that are found in unsalted nuts and seeds, fish (especially oily fish, such as salmon, trout, and herring, at least twice per week) and vegetable oils.

**Limit cholesterol intake to less than 300 mg per day, for most people.** If you have coronary heart disease or your LDL cholesterol level is 100 mg/dL or greater, limit your cholesterol intake to less than 200 milligrams a day. Some food groups may be beneficial in directly lowering cholesterol levels and include foods with plant sterol additives, high fiber foods like bran, oatmeal, and fruits like apples and pears, fish, nuts, and olive oil. Some of these foods like nuts and fruits are also high in calories, so moderation is always advisable.

**What other lifestyle interventions help lower cholesterol?**

**Weight loss and exercise are shown to decrease total cholesterol while increasing levels of HDL, the good cholesterol.** Smoking cessation decreases LDL levels plus smoking is a primary risk factor for heart disease and stroke. One drink of alcohol a day may help increase HDL levels (amongst other effects), but too much alcohol can damage the liver and increase the risk of elevated LDL. No physician should recommend alcohol as therapeutic strategy due to

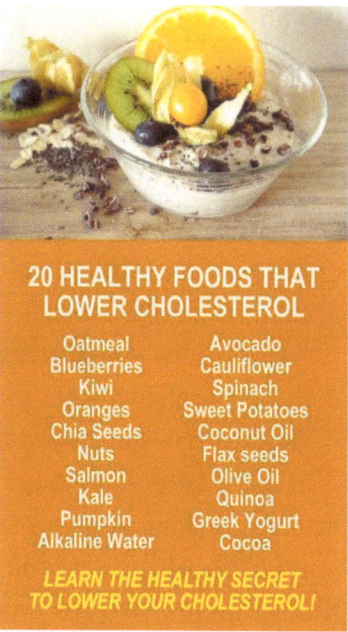

**20 HEALTHY FOODS THAT LOWER CHOLESTEROL**

| | |
|---|---|
| Oatmeal | Avocado |
| Blueberries | Cauliflower |
| Kiwi | Spinach |
| Oranges | Sweet Potatoes |
| Chia Seeds | Coconut Oil |
| Nuts | Flax seeds |
| Salmon | Olive Oil |
| Kale | Quinoa |
| Pumpkin | Greek Yogurt |
| Alkaline Water | Cocoa |

*LEARN THE HEALTHY SECRET TO LOWER YOUR CHOLESTEROL!*

the long term documented adverse side effects of sustained excess alcohol usage.

**There is no safe alcohol use level but there may be an ideal tolerated level for each person.** Alcohol at any level chronically also increases the risk of breast cancer, throat, liver, and colon/rectal cancers.

## What medications are available to treat high cholesterol?

**Seven major classes of drug classes are used to lower cholesterol levels:**

**Statins:** A variety of statin drugs are on the market including simvastatin (Zocor), atorvastatin (Lipitor), pravastatin (Pravachol), fluvastatin (Lescol), lovastatin (Mevacor), and rosuvastatin (Crestor). **These drugs primarily decrease LDL cholesterol.**

**Niacin:** Niaspan is the prescription form of niacin and decreases LDL and triglycerides as well as increases HDL cholesterol.

**Bile acid resins:** Cholestyramine (Questran) is a bile acid resin and decreases LDL.

**Fibric acid derivatives:** Fibric acid resins lower LDL and include gemfibrozil (Lopid) and fenofibrate (Tricor).

Statins are the only class of oral cholesterol lowering drugs that have been causally related to reducing the risk of heart attack, cardiovascular death, limb amputation, and stroke.

**PCSK9 inhibitors:** Alirocumab (Praluent) and evolocumab (Repatha) are two new medications called **PCSK9 inhibitors**, that are antibodies to a protein, PCSK9, a receptor for LDL, and are administered by monthly periodic subcutaneous skin injections. These drugs are indicated for treatment in patients who have had heart attack or stroke or have familial hypercholesterolemia and are taking maximum therapy, but continue to have high LDL cholesterol levels in their blood. These medicines have been proven to reduce cardiovascular death, strokes, unstable angina and myocardial infarctions (heart attacks) in those after an initial heart attack even after the LDL cholesterol has been intensively lowered using statin medications (**ODYSSEY OUTCOMES** and **FOURIER** trials). There also newer drugs that offer an alternative to statin therapy for those with moderate LDL elevations and **intolerance to statin therapy** due to side effects such as muscle pain, liver abnormalities, etc. One such drug is called Bempedoic acid (**Nexlitol** and can be taken in combination with an intestinal cholesterol absorption blocker called Ezetimibe (**Nexlizet.**

**Eicosapentaenoic acid (Icosapent Ethyl): VASCEPA**™ is icosapent ethyl (IPE), and is the only FDAapproved EPA and CV risk–reducing agent. IPE has undergone a proprietary purification process which has been approved and validated by the FDA. This process effectively removes LDLraising DHA, saturated fats, toxins, and other impurities, leaving only a single purified ingredient 96% plus pure Eicosapentaenoic acid (EPA). In 2019, the FDA designated this single purified ingredient IPE, a new chemical entity. approved the use of Vascepa™ (icosapent ethyl) as an adjunctive (secondary) therapy to reduce the risk of cardiovascular events among adults with elevated triglyceride levels (a type of fat in the blood) of 150 milligrams per deciliter or higher. Patients must also have either established cardiovascular disease or diabetes and two or more additional risk factors for cardiovascular disease.

Your physician will discuss what cholesterol medications are right for you based on your current and past medical history, your current health, and any other medications you are taking. These medications often need to be adjusted and monitored clinically using laboratory tests for liver and skeletal muscle damage for assessing side effects.

While all these medication groups may have a role in controlling cholesterol levels in association with diet, exercise, and smoking cessation, only statins, PCSK9 inhibitors and Vascepa have been shown to decrease the risk of heart attack and cardiovascular death.

Statin therapy may benefit patients with a history of heart attack, those with elevated blood LDL cholesterol levels or type two diabetes, and those with a 10year risk of heart disease greater than 7.5%. When monitoring how well statin therapy works, the goal for some individuals is no longer to reach a specific blood cholesterol level. Instead, patients with a high risk of heart disease will aim to decrease their cholesterol levels by 50% and those with a lesser risk will aim to lower their cholesterol levels by at least 30% to 50%. Everyone will need to discuss what levels are best for them with their physician. Remember some lipid lowering therapies such as statins **work in multiple "pleiotropic" ways** to reduce cardiovascular risks including lowering LDL cholesterol, and lowering inflammation in and stabilizing the vessel wall.

## 10 products to lower your increased cholesterol

### Oatmeal

Oatmeal contains a lot of fiber and promotes the metabolism and excretion of cholesterol. Other good sources of fiber – barley, beans, peas, lentil, fruits and vegetables, especially apples, dried plums, and raisins.

### Vegetable oils

These provide your body with healthy unsaturated fats and sterols which are the plant origin healthy equivalents of cholesterol. Other good sources – nuts and grains.

### Fatty sea fish

Salmon, mackerel, herring – these are the perfect source of Omega3 fatty acids. Why are natural Omega3 fatty acids so important? They prevent deposition of cholesterol in the walls of blood vessels. Other sources – codliver oil, seafood, linseed oil, tofu, almonds.

### Soy

Soy contains a lot of lecithins which help to maintain the right level of cholesterol. Other sources – egg yolks (but these also con – tain a lot of cholesterol, so it's better to get this from other products).

## Garlic

The active substance in garlic is allicin. Naturopathy considers garlic as one of the most effective substances to fight elevated cholesterol. Other sources of allicin are onion and leek.

## Artichoke essential oil

This has the ability to regulate and improve the levels of cholesterol and triglycerides.

## Evening primrose seeds oil

Evening primrose oil is an excellent source of unsaturated fats that improve the functioning of the blood circulation and control the level of cholesterol.t

## Dandelion

An extract of dandelion root has been used to improve liver function. The dandelion plant contains bioactive compounds that have been shown to reduce blood pressure, blood sugar and cholesterol in animal studies.

## Lucerne

This contains a lot of saponins that prevent the deposition of cholesterol in blood vessel walls.

## Useful dietary tips about cholesterol

- **Avoid saturated fats and trans fats.**
  Always carefully choose the products that you eat. Avoid the food that is contains a lot of saturated fats and substitute it with healthier, unsaturated fats. Try to reduce any and all dietary products of animal origin.
- **Eat more unsaturated fats.**
  Unsaturated fats are good for lowering the cholesterol level. Good products here are fish, most of the vegetable oils, avocado, and soy.
- **Go a little crazy with fruits and vegetables**
  Fruits and vegetables contain elements that can help you achieve the right level of cholesterol – mainly fiber and sterols. The most healthfriendly are – green leafy vegetables, squash, carrot, tomatoes, strawberry, plums, and blueberry. A little interesting saying about fruits and vegetables – the more colorful they are on your plate, the better they are for you. (Mediterranean Diet)
- **Avoid refined sugars and grains.**
  Whole grains are a good source of fiber. Try to include them in your diet as much as you can. Use wholegrain flour, brown rice, traditional, old school oatmeal.
- **Remember to count calories.**
  If you want to keep a diet that is healthy for your heart, you should count calories and be more aware of nutritional value of everything you eat.

- **Get over snacks and fast foods.**
  Try to not to eat between meals if you are really hungry – choose healthy snacks e.g. low sugar fruits and nuts. Remember to maximize healthy fats in your diet.

**Products to add to your diet: low-cholesterol**

**Peppers**

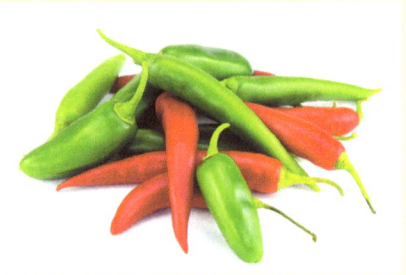

All kinds of peppers are good for you. It does not matter what color and how spicy they are. Consumption of peppers can have many advantages for your health. They lower cholesterol and blood pressure and can even improve the condition of your vessels. What is more, people that usually eat spicier food, consume less salt as an additive, which is always a good choice. The average size pepper has around 30 kcal, many antioxidants, and Vitamins – C and A. IDEA: Use spices (Basil Oregano, Chili peppers etc..) to reduce salt requirements for taste.

**Oats**

Do you want to lower your cholesterol eating breakfast? **Eat a bowl of oatmeal every morning**. Studies show that oats are the most effective grains when it comes to lowering the cholesterol level. Actually, oatmeal is not the only way to put oats in your diet. You can find many delicious meals based on oats – look ats especially in traditional recipes for soups and crunchy oatmeal bars. Barley and other whole grains.

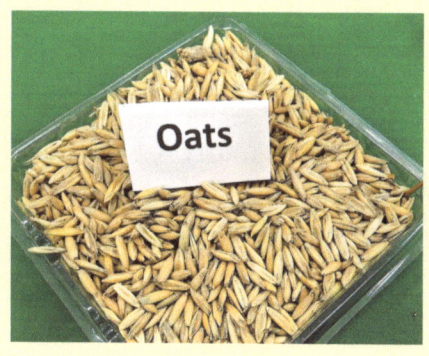

All the whole grain products are good as a part of a diet for people with heartrelated problems. **The biggest advantage is the high amount of soluble fiber.**

## Beans

**Beans are a great source of fiber.** It takes some time to be digested, so you would feel full for longer – it is good for people trying to lose some weight. Different kinds are available: white and red bean, peas, green Kate Dorosz beans, lentils, etc. There are also so many ways to prepare these.

## Eggplant

Nutritious tasty and a great source of fiber. Popular in the Mediterranean diet and cuisine, and healthy also!

## Nuts

A diet of almonds, walnuts, peanuts or any other kind of nuts is good for the heart. Just 2 servings a day can reduce your cholesterol by 5%. Nuts also have other nutrients that are good for heart health. Moreover, recently a Mediter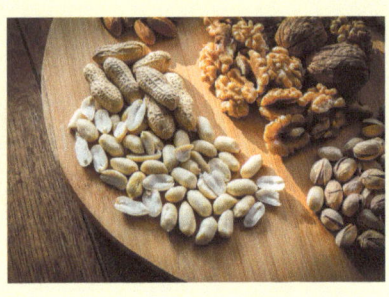ranean diet rich in olive oil, fruit, nuts, vegetables, and cereals along with a moderate intake of fish and poultry; a low intake of dairy products, red meat, processed meats, and sweets; and wine in moderation can reduce the incidence of major cardiovascular events compared with those who just follow a reducedfat diet. The amount and type of fats and other nutrients in the diet do matter.

## Vegetable oils

Using appropriate vegetable oils instead of saturated fats can significantly reduce your cholesterol level.

## Apples, grapes, citrus

These contain a lot of pectin (a kind of fiber) that is very effective in reducing cholesterol.

## Food with added sterols

Sterols have the ability to reduce the absorption of cholesterol. Some food companies are producing special lines of food with extra sterols, for example, margarine, granola bars, chocolate or orange juices.

## Soy

Consuming soy is often recommended as a good way to lower the cholesterol level. Studies suggest that eating 25g of soy protein daily may decrease the cholesterol by as much as 5%. You can find an excellent selection of soy products at every store.

## Fish

Eating fish once or twice a week can lower the cholesterol and protect your heart from several diseases. Try to eat fish instead of meat as much as you can.

## EXERCISE

To lower cholesterol and diminish cardiovascular risk, you have to utilize 3 strategies together– exercise, weight loss and a balanced diet. Let us focus on exercise. The most popular and effective way to achieve cardio
vascular fitness and protection according to multiple investigations is aerobic/ fitness exercises such as running

swimming cycling and jogging. One of the important things you need to accomplish if you are trying to fight elevated cholesterol is to lose some weight. Obesity is one of the causes of heart and vascular problems and 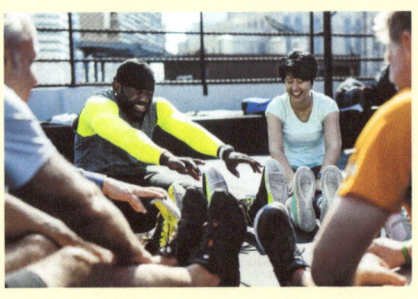 also it increases the body's tendency to accumulate more harmful cholesterol laden lipoproteins. The more you exercise, the more cholesterol is excreted from your body. Exercising also changes the size of atherogenic cholesterol (plaque causing) lipoproteins in the blood from small dense harmful LDL – cholesterol to more protective larger buoyant HDLcholesterol.

## How much should you exercise?

The exact amount and intensity of training is always a personal thing and should always be discussed with your doctor. Although, more is better only up to a point. However, the absolute minimum is 30 minutes daily. It does not have to be typical training. You can go for a walk, do some yoga, but also work in your garden... any physical activity will be good for you. Also, more intense training adopted gradually is the goal. Try to challenge yourself a little bit, to achieve better results. Dr. William Kraus states, that just mild training may not be sufficient when it comes to decreasing the blood cholesterol level. More strenuous exercise training regimens may yield incremental effects. Of course, any exercise is always better

# A Holistic Approach to Understanding...

than none, but... the more effort you put in it, the better results you can expect. Remember, it is all about your health, you must take control.

## How to begin?

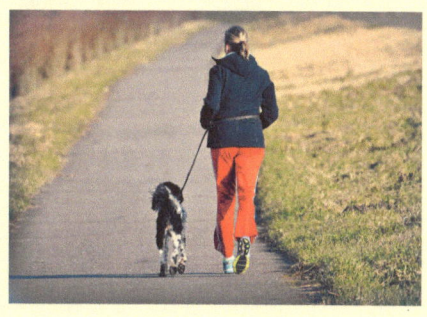

If you have never really exercised before, remember to talk about it with your doctor. Sometimes it is good to take a blood test and a physical examination before embarking on a new exercise program. Pick the activity that you can handle for 10 20 minutes without a break, at a sustainable intensity. Find the activity that you really like. Something, that it is a pleasure for you. Find a partner, somebody who would like to exercise with you, so you can motivate each other. It is always good to have a range of sporting interests, so you won't get bored, and you will exercise different groups of muscles.

## Chapter 5
# Healthy Heart and stress

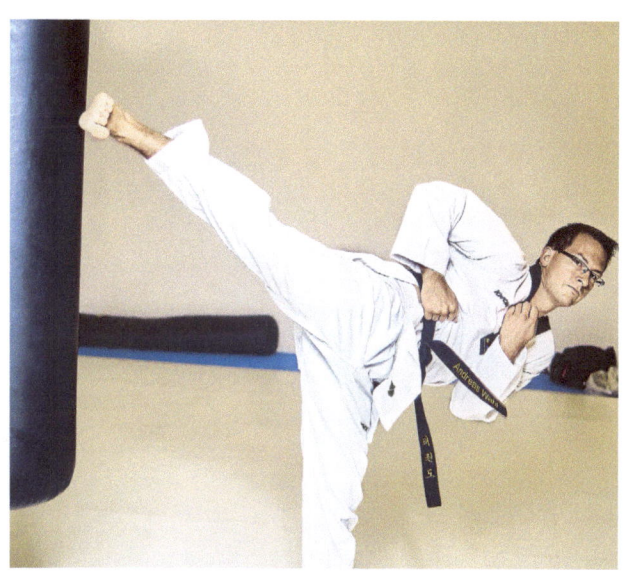

## Stress

When you get an unexpected bill, a dead car battery, divorce, death of a close one, or family trouble on your hands, are you like a cartoon character with steam shooting out of your ears or a cool cat who manages your stress calmly? Everyone feels stress in different ways and reacts to it in different ways. How much stress you experience and how you react to it, especially on a longterm basis, can lead to a wide vari – ety of health problems – and that's why it's critical to know how to handle stress.

## Stress and Your Heart

**Stress is toxic! Most heart attacks are due to coronary arteries being blocked by blood clots that form when plaques of cholesterol rupture.** The lack of blood flow through the blocked arteries results in heart muscle death, called a "heart attack." But over the past few years, physicians have come to recognize another form of heart attack. This unusual type of heart attack does not involve rupturing plaques or blocked blood vessels. It is called **takotsubo cardiomyopathy**, or "stress cardiomyopathy". Japanese doctors, who were the first to describe this condition, named it "takotsubo" because during this disorder, the heart takes on a distinctive shape that resembles a Japanese fishing pot used to trap an octo – pus! The disorder was commonly believed to be caused by sudden emotional stress, such as the death of a child, and to be far less harmful than a typical heart attack. For this reason, some have labeled this condition **"brokenheart syndrome."** More research is needed to determine how stress contributes to heart disease which is the leading cause of death in the Western and developing world. Stress can affect behaviors and risk factors that increase risk for heart disease: high blood pressure, high cholesterol levels, smoking, recreational drugs, physical inactivity and overeating. Some people may choose to drink too much alcohol or smoke cigarettes to "manage" their chronic stress, however these habits can increase blood pressure and damage vessel walls causing artery occlusion.

**Use of recreational drugs, alcohol, or tobacco to deal with stress is neither successful in the long term nor advisable.**

**Well known stress effects**
- Body aches and pains
- Decreased energy and disturbed sleep
- Feelings of anxiety, anger, and depression
- Impatience
- Forgetfulness

Your body's response to stress may be physical symptoms such as a headache, back strain, or stomach pains. Stress can also deplete your energy, destroy your sleep and make you feel irritable, forgetful and worse still leave you with a sense of being "out of control". **A stressful situation can set off a biological chain of events.** Your body releases the stress hormone adrenaline, a hormone that temporarily causes your breathing and heart rate to speed up and your blood pressure to rise. These reactions prepare you to deal with a threatening situation – the so called "fight or flight" response.

When stress is constant even at moderate levels, your body remains in high gear off and on for days or weeks at a time. Although the link between stress and heart disease isn't clear, chronic stress is very deleterious and may cause some people to drink too much alcohol and smoke which can increase your blood pressure and may damage the artery walls and heart muscle.

**Can managing stress reduce or prevent heart disease?**

Managing stress is a good idea for your overall health, and researchers are currently studying whether managing stress can prevent heart disease. Studies using psychosocial therapies – involving both psychological and social aspects – are promising in the prevention of a second heart attack. After a heart attack or stroke, people who feel depressed, anxious or overwhelmed by stress should talk to their doctor or other healthcare professionals. It is a fact that when patients develop depression after major illness e.g. a heart attack the outcomes are poor.

**What can you do about stress?**

**Exercising, maintaining a positive attitude, not smoking, not drinking too much coffee or other stimulants, enjoying a healthy diet and maintaining a healthy weight are good ways to deal with stress.** Medicines are helpful for many things, but usually not for stress. Some people take tranquilizers to calm stress down immediately, but it's far better in the long term to learn to manage your stress through relaxation or nonpharmacological stress management techniques (yoga, meditation). While stress can lead to anxiety feelings, the two are not the same condition. Anxiety can arise without any obvious stressful provocation, due to imbalance in certain brain chemical transmitters and is amenable to both pharmacologic and psychosocial therapies. Figuring out how stress pushes your buttons is an important step in dealing with it and preventing consequent depression and anxiety.

**When you are under stress, do you:**
- eat to calm down?
- speak and eat very fast?
- drink alcohol or smoke?
- rush around but do not get much done?
- work too much?
- procrastinate?
- sleep too little, too much or both?
- slow down?
- try to do too many things all at once?

Engaging in even one of these behaviors may mean that you are not dealing with stress effectively. If your stress is nonstop and unavoidable due to work or life circumstances, stress management classes can also help. Look for them at community colleges, rehab programs, in hospitals or by calling a therapist in your community.

People respond to stressful situations differently. Some react strongly to a situation. Others are relaxed and unconcerned. **Luckily, you can decrease the effect of stress on your body.** First, identify situations that cause stress. Although it is difficult, try to control your mental and physical reactions to these stressful situations.

### Get plenty of exercise

Exercise can help counteract the harmful effects of stress. For heart health, aim for at least 30 to 40 minutes, 4 to 5 days a week. Exercise can help to improve cardiovascular health by controlling weight, improving lipid levels (blood fats), and lowering blood pressure. Exercise has another benefit that lowers stress. **People who exercise have a reduced physical response to stress.** Their blood pressure and heart rates don't go up as high as people under stress who don't exercise. Regular exercise can also reduce the risk of depression, another risk factor for heart disease. Need exercise motivation? **Get a pedometer and try to walk 10,000 steps to 12,000 steps per day**. This may also help you maintain your weight. With a pedometer, you get instant feedback and credit for all you do, such as taking the stairs instead of the elevator.

### Build a strong support system

Research suggests that having a **strong social support network** like being married, having someone you can talk to and trust, or belonging to organizations or an organized religion can reduce your stress level and also your risk of heart disease. If you already have heart disease, this same network can help reduce your risk for heart attack. Having at least one person you can rely on takes a heavy burden off you and provides comfort. A strong support system helps you take better care of yourself, too. Research shows that a lack of social support increases the chance of engaging in unhealthy behaviors like smoking, eating highfat foods, and drinking too much alcohol.

**Seek treatment for constant depression or anxiety**

**Depression and anxiety** can increase your risk of dying from heart disease if you already have it. In one study, people were asked whether they had felt so sad, discouraged, or hopeless during the past month that they had wondered if anything was worthwhile. Those who answered yes had more than twice the risk for coronary artery disease. **Many studies suggest that longterm anxiety can increase the risk for sudden cardiac death.** To reduce your anxiety level, try activities that reduce stress like yoga, walking meditation, traditional meditation, guided imagery, or other methods. Look for classes in your area. Talk with your provider if you have feelings of depression or anxiety and ask about medicines and other therapies that may help.

**Reduce stress from work**

Studies show having a demanding job that offers you few opportunities to make decisions or provides little reward can increase your risk for heart disease. Stress at work becomes even more of a problem when you do not have a strong support system, or if you have longterm anxiety. If you cannot find a different position within your company, do what you can to gain control over your environment.

**Try to take some time every day away from work.**

Do something that is relaxing and that you enjoy. It may be reading, walking, or deep breathing. Your employer may offer an employee assistance program (EAP) to help you manage stress and anxiety. **A counselor can help recommend strategies to help you lower your workrelated stress.**

**4 ways to manage stress and help your heart**

**Stay positive.** People with heart disease who maintain an upbeat attitude are less likely to die of it than those who are more negative. **Just having a good laugh can help your heart.** Laughter, joy and happiness really is the best medicine. Laughter has been found to lower levels of stress hormones, reduce inflammation in the arteries, and increase "good" HDL cholesterol.

**Meditate**. This practice of inwardfocused thought and controlled measured deep breathing has been shown to reduce heart disease risk factors such as high blood pressure. Anyone can learn to meditate. Just take a few minutes to sit somewhere quiet, close your eyes, and focus on your breathing. Yoga and prayer can also relax the mind and body **Exercise.**

Every time you are physically active, whether you take a walk or play tennis, your body releases moodboosting chemicals called endorphins. Exercising not only melts away stress, but it also protects against heart disease by lowering your blood pressure, strengthening your heart muscle, and helping you maintain a healthy weight.

**Unplug.** It is impossible to escape stress when it follows you everywhere. **Cut the cord. Avoid emails and TV news.**

Take time each day–even if it's for just 10 or 15 minutes– to escape from the world. Find your own path to stress relief. Take a hot bath, listen to music, or read a book. Any technique is effective if it works for you...

## A SMART way to ease stress

A range of programs are available to help people enhance their quality of life and cope with different medical conditions. Stress Management and Resilience Training (SMART) program teach selfcare practices that help buf – fer daily stress and foster resilience – the ability to cope with stress.

During individual and group sessions, people learn about stress and its connection to physical or emotional problems. The program also emphasizes importance of healthy eating, restorative sleep, and physical activity. One key focus is learning a variety of techniques to elicit the relaxation response, which is the opposite of the stress response.

First described in the 1970s at Harvard Medical School by cardiologist Dr. Herbert Benson, the relaxation response can be elicited in many ways, including meditation or repetitive prayer.

**You can evoke this calming response with two simple steps:**

**Step 1**: Choose a calming focus. Good examples are your breath, a sound ("om"), a short prayer, or a positive word (such as "relax" or "peace") or phrase ("breathing in calm, breathing out tension"; "I am relaxed"). Repeat this aloud or silently as you inhale or exhale.

**Step 2:** Let go and relax. Do not worry about how you're doing. When you notice your mind has wandered, simply take a deep breath or say to yourself "refocus, refocus" and gently return your attention to your focus. Practicing these two steps for 10 to 20 minutes a day may help reduce the effects of stress on your body.

Katarzyna Dorosz

## HERBS

**Lavender**

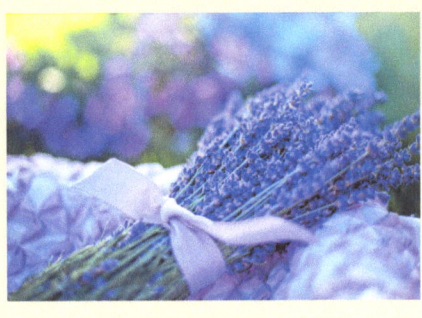

Lavender is a wellknown Mediterranean herb, especially popular in Europe. Commonly employed as a medicine in ancient Egypt, Greece, Rome, and Arabic countries, lavender was used in essential oils for aromatic baths, as a soap, but also for the mummification process. Its name comes from Latin "lavare" that means "bath". Later, in medieval times, it was used as a medication and for some religious purposes. Fresh lavender can be used as a tea great for calming and lessening pain. It can also be good to prevent fainting. It is a good remedy for sore throat and joint pain in joints. It can be used to cure inflammation, cuts, and scrapes. **Lavender essential oils and candles are a great adjunct for relaxation.**

**Lemon balm (Melissa officinalis, balm mint)**

Lemon balm originally comes from Europe and North Africa. People have been using it since ancient times. Originally used as part of a "longevity elixir", it was well known for its revitalizing features, and then later, its medicinal properties were exploited for relief of pain, anxiety, and depression. It was even used for bites of bugs, scorpions, and dogs.

Lemon balm is said to soothe symptoms of stress, help you to relax, and boost your mood. One study found that taking lemon balm eased the negative mood effects of laboratoryinduced psychological stress. Participants who took lemon balm selfreported an increased sense of calmness and reduced feelings of agitation. Although this was a doubleblind, placebo – controlled study, it had a small sample size of 18 people. Further research is needed to elaborate on these findings.

**How to use:** Take 300 milligrams (mg) of lemon balm in capsule form twice a day. You can take a single dose of 600 mg in acute episodes of stress.

Lemon balm tea indeed is an "elixir of longevity". It has so many different proven features. Excellent as a cold and flu treatment, it can be used to lower blood pressure, treat insomnia and relieve indigestion. Because of its antianxiety and mild antidepressant functions (rosmarinic acid component), it can be used for anxiety, depression, and to reduce stress, and tension. Lemon balm is able to enhance heart function by relaxing the blood vessels and lowering the blood pressure

## Saffron

Saffron originally come from Italy but was also popular in India, Turkey, China, and Iran. It has a unique flavor and color – can be used as a potent natural food coloring. Saffron is well known

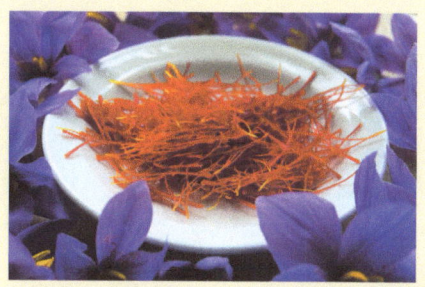

for its medicinal functions – it is a good antioxidant, immunity enhancer and is antiinflammatory. It also has anticancer properties! Saffron is traditionally used because of its antiseptic properties.

**Valerian root**

Commonly used over the centuries for its calming and relaxing features, it has found an established place both in traditional and conventional medicine. It reduces menopausal symptoms and can reduce the severity and frequency of hot flashes in post – menopausal women. Valerian can cause **withdrawal symptoms** if discontinued suddenly and does interact to boost harmful side effects with alcohol, benzodiazepines, barbiturates, and other antidepressant medications.

**EXERCISES**

**Exercising is one of the bestknown ways to reduce stress and anxiety.** When you are working out your body produces and releases endorphins, the "hormones of joy". These help you feel better, relaxed, and more ready to face any of life's challenges especially after a good training work out. What are the best ways to relax by working out? Cardiovascular ("Cardio") workouts Everything that elevates your working heart rate by at least a moderate sustainable level and that expends calories would work here – jogging, dancing, spinning, cycling, roller skating. Really, whatever you like, just make it intermittently intense and sustainable. Exercise is the instant "fix" and can make you feel better and energized – both physically and mentally. No side effects and minimal cost to you!

**Remember, if you want to start a really intense physical activity particularly for the first time, please discuss it first with your physician.**

## Yoga

Yoga in both its meditative spiritual and physical forms is an excellent form of relaxation. As a mix of exercise, breathing, and meditation it can really help you **relax, calm down and spiritually rejuvenate**. It is the ultimate activity for your body and mind. It can also help you to keep your balance and homeostasis – a fundamental basis of good health.

## Tai chi

Similarly, Tai Chi can be a good relaxation technique even for the elderly, if you do not make it too intense. Slow, precise movement and calm breathing can help you feel better after a stressful situation. Tai Chi has many other advantages for your heart and overall health. It's also one of the sports, that after a few lessons with an instructor, you can continue by yourself, whenever and wherever you want. Just remember about keeping it appropriate, not too high a level of intensity.

Katarzyna Dorosz

**Pilates**

Pilates is a good training to enhance body flexibility, strength endurance and overall capability. Another good sport for stress. It can also help you to tone muscles, build muscular strength and promote weight loss.

**Tennis**

Take your family or friends and go play together. Pick tennis, or any other sport you can play in a group. Soccer, volleyballwhatever you would like. Exercising and sweating in good company makes it easier and even more enjoyable. After all, the more fun you have – the better you feel.

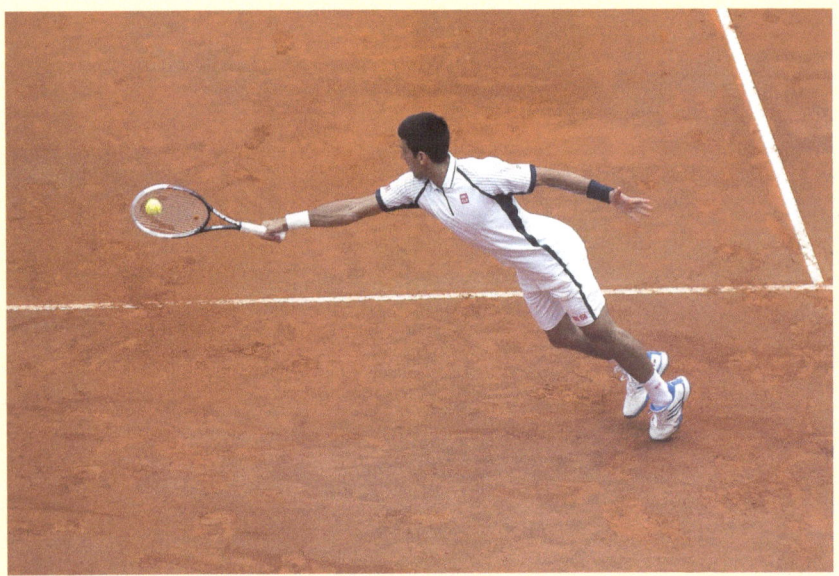

# Chapter 6
# Prostate

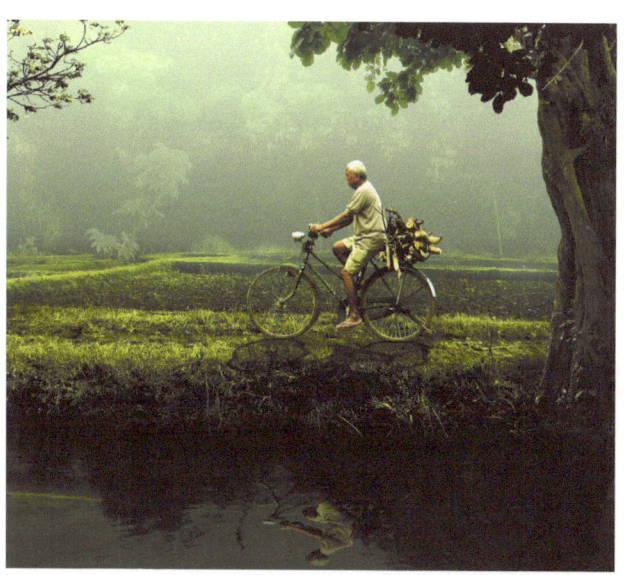

## Prostate health

The prostate gland has an important job in males: it produces a thick, milkywhite fluid that becomes part of the semen, the liquid ejaculated during sexual activity. The gland is actually usually rather small– about the size of a walnut or golf ball–but its location virtually guarantees problems if something goes awry. The prostate gland is located just below the bladder and in front of the rectum. It also wraps around the upper part of the urethra, the tube that carries urine from the bladder out of the body.

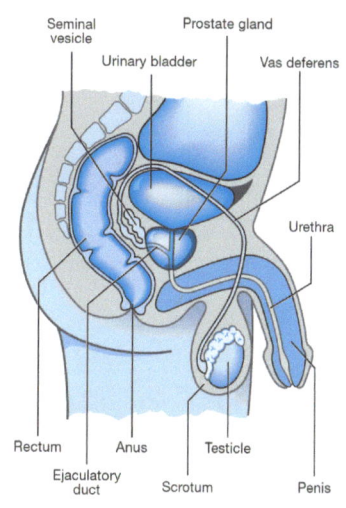

**Prostate problems can affect urination and sexual function.**

### The prostate is prone to three main conditions:

**Prostatitis:** infection or inflammation of the prostate. Prostatitis can cause burning or painful urination, the urgent need to urinate, trouble urinating, difficult or painful ejaculation, and pain in the area between the scrotum and rectum (known as the perineum) or in the lower back.

**Benign prostatic hyperplasia (BPH):** A process of agingrelated enlargement of the prostate gland. (BPH) can cause the prostate to compress the urethra and slow or even stop the flow of urine, in much the same way that bending

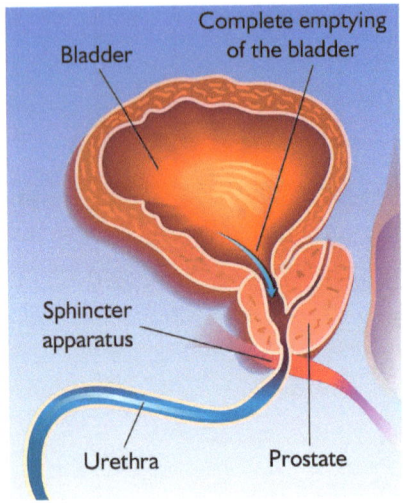 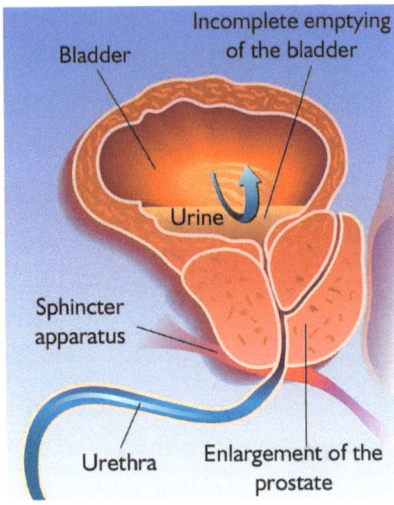

a garden hose chokes off the flow of water. BPH affects about threequarters of men over age 60.

**Prostate cancer:** the growth of cancerous cells inside the prostate, which may break out of the gland and affect other parts of the body. In the United States, about 1 man in 7 will be diagnosed with prostate cancer during his lifetime. It occurs mainly in older men.

**How the Prostate Changes with Age**

Because the prostate gland tends to grow larger with age, it may squeeze the urethra and cause problems in passing urine. Sometimes men in their 30s and 40s may begin to have these urinary symptoms and need medical attention. For others, symptoms aren't noticeable until much later in life. An infection or a tumor can also make the prostate larger.

## Be sure to tell your doctor if you have any of the following urinary symptoms:

- Are passing urine more frequently during the day
- Have an urgent need to pass urine
- Have weak urine flow that starts and stops
- Feel burning when you pass urine
- Need to get up frequently during the night to pass urine

## Growing older raises your risk of prostate problems

The three most common prostate problems are inflammation (prostatitis), enlarged prostate (BPH, or benign prostatic hyperplasia), and prostate cancer. **Having prostatitis or an enlarged prostate does not necessarily increase your risk of prostate cancer.**

**Prostate Changes That Are Not Cancer Prostatitis**

Prostatitis is an **inflammation of the prostate** gland that may result from a bacterial infection. It affects at least half of all men at some time during their lives. Having this condition does not increase your risk of any other prostate disease.

## Symptoms of prostatitis

- Trouble passing urine
- A burning or stinging feeling or pain when passing urine

- Strong, frequent urge to pass urine, even when there is only a small amount of urine passed
- Chills and high fever
- Low back pain or body aches
- Pain low in the belly, groin, or behind the scrotum
- Rectal pressure or pain
- Urethral discharge with bowel movements
- Genital and rectal throbbing
- Sexual problems and loss of sex drive
- Painful ejaculation (sexual climax)

## Types of Prostatitis and Treatments

### Acute bacterial prostatitis

This condition is caused by a bacterial infection and comes on suddenly (acutely). Symptoms include severe chills and fever. There is often blood in the urine. **PSA levels** (see PSA test) may be higher than normal. You must go to the doctor's office or emergency room for treatment if prostatitis occurs. It is the least common of the four types, yet it is the easiest to diagnose and treat. Most cases can be cured with a **high dose of antibiotic**s, taken for 7 to 14 days, and then lower doses for several weeks. You may also need drugs to help with pain or discomfort. If the PSA level was high, it will likely return to normal once the infection is cleared up. This requires follow up with a physician.

## Chronic bacterial prostatitis

Also caused by bacteria, this type of prostatitis does not come on suddenly, but it can be bothersome. The only symptom you may have is bladder infections that keep coming back. The cause may be a defect in the prostate that lets bacteria collect in the urinary tract. Antibiotic treatment over a longer period of time is best for this type. Treatment lasts from 4 to 12 weeks. This treatment clears up about 60 percent of cases. Longterm, lowdose antibiotics may help relieve symptoms in cases that Are difficult to clear up.

## Chronic prostatitis or chronic pelvic pain syndrome

This disorder is the most common but least understood type of prostatitis. Found in men of any age from late teens to the elderly, its symptoms can come and go without warning. There can be pain or discomfort in the groin or bladder area. Infectionfighting white blood cells are often present, even though no bacteria can be found. There are several different treatments for this problem, based on your symptoms. These include antiinflammatory medications and other pain control treatments, such as warm baths. Medicines, such as alphablockers, may also be given. Alphablockers relax muscle tissue in the prostate to make urine flow easier. Some men are treated with antibiotics in case the symptoms are caused by an undetected infection.

Dr. Sanjay Srivatsa

## Asymptomatic (No symptoms) inflammatory prostatitis

You do not have symptoms with this condition. It is often found when you are undergoing tests for other conditions, such as to determine the cause of infertility or to look for prostate cancer. If you have this form of prostatitis, your PSA test may show a higher number than normal. Men with this condition are usually not treated, but a repeat PSA test will usually be done if the PSA number is high.

## Enlarged Prostate (BPH)

BPH stands for benign prostatic hyperplasia. Benign means "not cancer," and hyperplasia means abnormal cell growth. The result here is that the prostate becomes enlarged. BPH is not linked to cancer and does not increase your risk of get‑ting prostate cancer–yet the symptoms for BPH and prostate cancer can be similar.

## Symptoms of BPH

- Trouble starting a urine stream, or the urine flow is no more than a dribble
- Passing urine often, especially at night
- Feeling constantly that the bladder has not fully emptied
- A strong or sudden urge to pass urine
- Weak or slow urine stream
- Stopping and starting again several times while passing urine (hesitancy)
- Pushing or straining to begin passing urine

At its worst, BPH can lead to a weak bladder, backflow of urine causing bladder or kidney infections, complete blockage in the flow of urine and kidney failure. The prostate gland is about the size of a walnut when a man is in his 20s. By the time he is 40, it may have grown slightly larger, to the size of an apricot. By age 60, it may be the size of a lemon. The enlarged prostate can press against the bladder and the urethra. This can slow down or block urine flow. Some men might find it hard to start a urine stream, even though they feel the need to go. Once the urine stream has started, it may be hard to stop. Men sometimes feel like they need to pass urine all the time, or they are awakened during sleep with the sudden need to pass urine. Early BPH symptoms take many years to turn into bothersome problems. These early symptoms are a cue to see your doctor.

**Treatments for BPH**

Some men with BPH eventually find their symptoms to be bothersome enough to need treatment. BPH cannot be cured, but drugs or surgery can often relieve its symptoms. Talk with your doctor about the best choice for you. Your symptoms may change over time, so be sure to tell your doctor about any new changes.

**Watchful waiting**

Men with mild symptoms of BPH who do not find them bothersome often choose this approach. Watchful waiting

means getting annual checkups. Treatment is started only if symptoms become too much of a problem. If you choose watchful waiting, these simple steps may help lessen your symptoms:
- Limit drinking in the evening, especially drinks with alcohol or caffeine.
- Empty your bladder all the way when you pass urine.
- Use the restroom often. Do not wait for long periods without passing urine.
- Some medications can make BPH symptoms worse, such as:
- Overthecounter cold and cough medicines (especially antihistamines)
- Tranquilizers
- Antidepressants
- Blood pressure medication.

### Drug Therapy

Many American men with **mild to moderate BPH symptoms** have chosen prescription drugs over surgery since the early 1990s. **Two main types of drugs are used.** One type relaxes muscles guarding the urine flow through the prostate, and the other type shrinks the volume of the prostate gland. Some evidence shows that taking both drugs together may work best to keep BPH symptoms from getting worse.

**Alphablockers** are drugs that help relax muscles near the prostate to relieve pressure and let urine flow more freely, but they do not shrink the size of the prostate. For many men, these drugs can improve urine flow and reduce the symptoms of BPH within days. Possible side effects include low BP, dizziness, headache, and fatigue.

**5 alphareductase inhibitors** are drugs that help shrink the prostate. They relieve symptoms by blocking the activity of an enzyme known as 5alpha reductase. This enzyme changes the male hormone testosterone into dihydrotestosterone (DHT), which stimulates prostate growth. When the action of 5alpha reductase is blocked, DHT production is lowered and prostate growth slows. This helps shrink the prostate, reduce blockage, and limit the need for surgery.

Taking these drugs can help increase urine flow and reduce your symptoms. You must continue to take these drugs to prevent symptoms from coming back. **5alpha reductase inhibitors can cause the following side effects in a small percentage of men including: decreased interest in sex, trouble getting or keeping an erection, and smaller amount of semen with ejaculation.**

It is important to note that taking **these drugs may lower your PSA test number.** There is also evidence that these drugs lower the risk of developing prostate cancer, but whether they can help lower the risk of dying from prostate cancer is still unclear.

## Surgery

The number of prostate surgeries has gone down over the years. But operations for BPH are still among the most common surgeries for American men. Surgery is used when symptoms are severe, or drug therapy has not worked well. Be sure to discuss options with your physician and ask about the potential short and longterm benefits and risks associated with each procedure.

## Types of surgery for BPH

### TURP (transurethral resection of the prostate)

The most common surgery for BPH, TURP accounts for 90 percent of all BPH surgeries. The doctor passes an instrument through the urethra and trims away extra prostate tissue. A spinal block (anesthesia) is used to numb the area. Tis – sue is sent to the laboratory to check for prostate cancer. **TURP generally avoids the two main dangers linked to another type of surgery called open prostatectomy** (complete removal of the prostate gland through a cut in the lower abdomen): including **incontinence and/or impotence**. However, TURP can have serious side effects, such as bleeding. In addition, men may have to stay in the hospital and need a urinary catheter for a few days after surgery.

### TUIP (transurethral incision of the prostate)

This surgery, which is like TURP, is used on slightly enlarged prostate glands. The surgeon places one or two small cuts in the prostate. This relieves pressure without trimming away tissue. It has a low risk of side effects. Like TURP, this treatment helps with urine flow by widening the urethra.

### TUNA (transurethral needle ablation)

Radio waves are used to burn away excess prostate tissue. TUNA helps with urine flow, relieves symptoms, and may have fewer side effects than TURP. Most men need a catheter to drain urine for a period of time after the procedure.

**TUMT (transurethral microwave thermotherapy)**. Microwaves sent through a catheter are used to destroy excess prostate tissue. This can be an option for men who should not have major surgery because they also have other medical problems.

**TUVP** (transurethral electro evaporation of the prostate)
An electrical current is used to vaporize prostate tissue.
**Laser surgery.** The doctor passes a laser fiber through the urethra into the prostate, using a cystoscope, and then delivers several bursts of laser energy. The laser energy destroys prostate tissue and helps improve urine flow. Like TURP, laser surgery requires anesthesia. One advantage of laser surgery over TURP is that laser surgery causes little blood loss. The recovery period for laser surgery may be shorter too. **However, laser surgery may not be as effective on larger prostates. Open prostatectomy.** This may be the only option in rare cases, such as when the obstruction is severe, the prostate is very large, or other procedures are not feasible.

General anesthesia or a spinal block is used, and a catheter remains in place for 3 to 7 days after the surgery. This surgery carries the highest risk of postoperative complications. Tissue is sent to the laboratory to check for prostate cancer.

**Prostate Cancer**

Prostate cancer means that cancer cells form in the tis – sues of the prostate. Prostate cancer tends to grow slowly compared with most other cancers. Cell changes may begin 10, 20, or even 30 years before a tumor gets big enough to cause symptoms. Eventually, cancer cells may spread (metastasize). By the time symptoms appear, the cancer may already be advanced.

By age 50, very few men have symptoms of prostate cancer, yet some precancerous or cancer cells may be present. **More than half of all American men have some cancer in their prostate glands by the age of 80.** Most of these cancers never pose a problem. They may never cause symptoms or become a serious threat to health.

### Symptoms of Prostate Cancer
- Trouble passing urine
- Frequent urge to pass urine, especially at night
- Weak or interrupted urine stream
- Pain or burning when passing urine
- Blood in the urine or semen
- Painful ejaculation
- Nagging pain in the back, hips, or pelvis

Prostate cancer can spread to the lymph nodes of the pelvis. Or it may spread throughout the body. It tends to spread to the bones. Bone pain, especially in the back, can be a symptom of advanced prostate cancer.

### Risk Factors for Prostate Cancer

Some risk factors have been linked to prostate cancer. A risk raises your chance of developing disease. Having one or more risk factors does not mean that you will get prostate cancer. It just means that your risk of the disease is greater.

### Age

Men who are 50 or older have a higher risk of prostate cancer.

### Race

**African American men have the highest risk of prostate cancer–the disease tends to start at younger ages and grows faster than in men of other races.** After African – American men, prostate cancer is most common among white men, followed by Hispanic and Native American men. AsianAmerican men have the lowest rates of prostate cancer.

### Family history

Men whose fathers or brothers have had prostate cancer have a 2 to 3 times higher risk of prostate cancer than men who do not have a family history of the disease. A man who has 3 immediate family members with prostate cancer has about 10 times the risk of a man who does not have a family history of prostate cancer. The younger a man's relatives are when they have prostate cancer, the greater his risk for developing the disease. Prostate cancer risk also appears to be slightly higher for men from families with a history of breast cancer.

## Diet

The risk of prostate cancer may be higher for men who eat highfat diets.

## Prostate Cancer Screening

Screening means testing for cancer before you have any symptoms. A screening test may help find cancer at an early stage when it is less likely to have spread and may be easier to treat or cure. By the time symptoms appear, the cancer may have already started to spread. The most useful screening tests are those that have been proven to lower a person's risk of dying from cancer. Doctors do not yet know whether prostate cancer screening lowers the risk of dying from prostate cancer. Therefore, large research studies, with thousands of men, are now going on to study prostate cancer screening. The National Cancer Institute is studying the combination of **PSA testing and Digital Rectal Examination (DRE)** as a way to achieve more accurate predictive information.

Although some people feel it is best to treat any cancer that is found, including cancers found through screening, prostate cancer treatment can cause serious and sometimes permanent side effects. Some doctors are concerned that many men whose cancer is detected by screening are being treated–and experiencing side effects–unnecessarily.

Talk with your doctor about your risk of prostate cancer and your need for screening tests.

## Tests Used to Check the Prostate

Your personal medical history also includes any risk factors, pain, fever, or trouble passing urine. You may be asked to give a urine sample for testing.

### Digital Rectal Exam (DRE)

The digital rectal exam is a standard way to check the prostate. With a gloved and lubricated finger, your doctor feels the prostate from the rectum. The test lasts about 1015 seconds. **This exam checks for:**
The size, firmness, and texture of the prostate
Any hard areas, lumps, or growth spreading beyond the prostate, and
Any pain caused by touching or pressing the prostate.
The DRE allows the doctor to feel only one side of the prostate. A PSA test is another way to help your doctor check the health of your prostate.

### PSA (ProstateSpecific Antigen) Test

**Many physicians use the PSA test along with a DRE to help detect prostate cancer in men age 50 and older.** PSA is a protein made by prostate cells. It is normally secreted into ducts in the prostate, where it helps make semen, but sometimes it leaks into the blood. When PSA is in the blood, it can be measured with a blood test called the PSA test. In prostate cancer, more PSA gets into the blood than is normal.

However, a high PSA blood level is not proof of cancer, and many other things can cause a falsepositive test result. For example, blood PSA levels are often increased in men with prostatitis or BPH. Any activity that pressurizes the prostate glandincluding riding a bicycle, or having a DRE, ejaculation within the past 24 hours, a prostate biopsy, or prostate surgerymay all increase PSA levels.

Also, some prostate glands naturally produce more PSA than others. PSA levels go up with age. **African American men tend to have higher PSA levels in general than men of other races.** And some drugs, such as finasteride and dutasteride, can cause a man's PSA level to go down. PSA tests are often used to follow men after prostate cancer treatment to check for signs of cancer recurrence. It is not yet known for certain whether PSA testing to screen for prostate cancer can reduce a man's risk of dying from the disease. Researchers are working to learn more about the PSA test's ability to help doctors tell the difference between prostate cancer and benign prostate problems, and the best thing to do if a man has a high PSA level. For now, physicians use serial PSA readings over time as a guide to see if more followup or investigation is needed.

**PSA test results**

PSA levels are measured in terms of the amount of PSA per volume of fluid tested. Doctors often use a value of 4 nanograms (ng) or higher per milliliter of blood as a sign that further tests, such as a prostate biopsy, are needed. Your doctor may monitor your **PSA velocity**, which means the rate of change in your PSA level over time. **Rapid increases in PSA readings may suggest cancer.** If you have a mildly elevated PSA level, you and your doctor may choose to do PSA tests on a scheduled basis and watch for any change in the PSA velocity.

**Free PSA test**

This test is used for men who have higher PSA levels. The standard PSA test measures total PSA, which includes both PSA that is attached, or bound, to other proteins and PSA that is free, or not bound. The free PSA test measures free PSA only. **Free PSA is linked to benign prostate conditions, such as BPH, whereas bound PSA is linked to cancer.** The percentage of free PSA can help tell what kind of prostate problem you have.

If both total PSA and free PSA are higher than normal (high percentage of free PSA), this suggests BPH rather than cancer. **If total PSA is high but free PSA is not (low percent – age of free PSA), cancer is more likely.** More testing, such as a biopsy, should be done. You and your doctor should talk about your personal risk and free PSA results. Then you can decide together whether to have followup biopsies and, if so, how often. There is no categorical PSA level below which a man can be assured of having no risk of prostate cancer nor above which a biopsy should automatically be performed. A man's decision to have a prostate biopsy requires a thoughtful discussion with his physician, considering not only the PSA level, but also his other risk factors, his overall health status, and how he perceives the risks and benefits of early detection.

## Prostate Biopsy

If your symptoms or test results suggest prostate cancer, your doctor will refer you to a specialist (a urologist) for a prostate biopsy. For a biopsy, small tissue samples are taken directly from the prostate. Your doctor will take samples from several areas of the prostate gland. This can help lower the chance of missing any areas of the gland that may have cancer cells. Like other cancers, prostate cancer can be diagnosed only by looking at tissue under a microscope. Most men who have biopsies after prostate cancer screening exams do not have cancer.

A positive test result after a biopsy means prostate cancer is present. A pathologist will check your biopsy sample for cancer cells and will give it a **Gleason score. The Gleason score ranges from 2 to 10 and describes how likely it is that a tumor will spread.** The lower the number, the less aggressive the tumor is and the less likely it will spread. Treatment options depend on the stage (or extent) of the cancer (stages range from 1 to 4), Gleason score, PSA level, and your age and general health. This information will be available from your doctor and is listed on your pathology report.

> "What can I eat to reduce my risk
> of developing prostate cancer?"

This is one of the most common questions physicians hear from men concerned about prostate health. Undoubtedly, many hope that their doctor will rattle off a list of foods guaranteed to shield them from disease. Although some foods have been linked with reduced risk of prostate cancer, proof that they really work is lacking, at least for now.

**Aim for a healthy eating pattern**

Instead of focusing on specific foods, dietitians, physicians, and researchers tout an overall pattern of healthy eating – and healthy eating is easier than you might think.

Here are what experts recommend:

- **Eat at least five servings of fruits and vegetables every day.** Go for those with deep, bright color.
- **Choose wholegrain bread instead of white bread**, and choose wholegrain pasta and cereals.
- **Limit your consumption of red meat**, including beef, pork, lamb, and goat, and processed meats, such as bologna and hot dogs. Fish, skinless poultry, beans, and eggs are healthier sources of protein.
- **Choose healthful fats**, such as olive oil, nuts (almonds, wal – nuts, pecans), and avocados. Limit saturated fats from dairy and other animal products. Avoid partially hydrogenated fats (trans fats), which are in many fast foods and packaged foods.

- **Avoid sugarsweetened drinks**, such as sodas and many
- fruit juices. Eat sweets as an occasional treat.
- **Cut down on salt.** Choose foods low in sodium by reading and comparing food labels. Limit the use of canned, pro – cessed, and frozen foods.
- **Watch portion sizes.** Eat slowly and stop eating when you are full.

Having a low blood level of vitamin D may be linked to a higher risk of developing some cancers, suggests a study published in the British Medical Journal BMJ. However, taking extra vitamin D to raise already normal levels does not appear to offer more protection. Vitamin D is made by the skin from sunlight exposure and can also be obtained through forti- fied foods like cereal and milk, as well as from supplements. Researchers analyzed data from the Japan Public Health Center based Prospective Study, involving 33,736 people ages 40 to 69. The people gave blood samples and were classed into four groups, ranging from the lowest to highest levels of vita – min D. They were then monitored for an average of 16 years, during which time 3,301 new cases of cancer were recorded among the participants. After adjusting for sever- al known cancer risk factors, such as age, weight, physical activity, smoking, alcohol intake, and dietary factors, the re- searchers found that **high levels of vitamin D were associ- ated with a 20% lower relative risk of cancer in both men and women compared with low vitamin D levels.** Higher vitamin D levels appeared to offer the clearest benefit for reducing liver cancer risk, especially for men. The researchers found no link between high vitamin D levels and lung or prostate cancer. It's not clear how vitamin D may lower cancer risk, but certain factors may explain the association. For instance, previous research has suggested **vitamin D has an antiinflammatory effect and may interfere with cancer cell pathways**. Also, people who tend to live healthier lifestyles are outside more often and thus are exposed to more vitamin D–generating sunlight. The researchers also noted that there appears to be a ceiling to vitamin D's influence against cancer, and that increasing a person's blood vitamin D level above 20 nanograms per milliliter, which is the amount considered adequate for bone and overall health, may not offer further benefits.

### Stay active and Loose Excess weight

In addition to eating a healthy diet, you should stay active. Regular exercise pares down your risk of developing some deadly problems, including heart disease, stroke, and certain types of cancer. And although relatively few studies have directly assessed the impact of exercise on prostate health, those that have been done have concluded, for the most part, that **exercise is beneficial.**

For example: Based on questionnaires completed by more than 30,000 men in the Health Professionals Followup Study, researchers found an inverse relationship between physical activity and BPH symptoms. Simply put, **men who were more physically active were less likely to suffer from BPH**. Even low – to moderateintensity physical activity, such as walking regularly at a moderate pace, yielded benefits for BPH. Using data from the Health Professionals Followup Study, researchers also examined the relationship between erectile dysfunction (ED) and exercise. They found that men who ran for an hour and a half or did three hours of rigorous outdoor work per week were 20% less likely to develop ED than those who didn't exercise at all. More physical activity conferred a greater benefit. Interestingly, regardless of the level of exercise, men who were overweight or obese had a greater risk of ED than men with an ideal body mass index, or BMI.

Italian researchers randomly assigned 231 sedentary men with chronic prostatitis to one of two exercise programs for 18 weeks: aerobic exercise, which included brisk walking, or nonaerobic exercise, which included leg lifts, situps, and stretching. Each group exercised three times a week. At the end of the trial, men in both groups felt better, but those in the **aerobic exercise group** experienced significantly less discomfort, anxiety and depression, and improved quality of life.

## Natural Products that promote prostate health

### Pygeum (African Plum extract)

Pygeum contains a lot of fatty acids and sterols e.g. beta-sitosterol, compounds that have potent antioxidant and anti – inflammatory actions on the genitourinary tract. 100200mg of pygeum extract daily can significantly decrease the symptoms of BPH (prostatism).

### Saw Palmetto

Saw Palmetto is one of the most popular herbal products used by the lay public as an adjunctive treatment for BPH. It has the ability to reduce prostatism symptoms and decrease the amount of produced testosterone (which stimulates prostatic tissue growth).

### ZiShen Pill

This pill is a mix of three herbs including Chinese cinnamon. It has been used since ancient times and is very popular in Chinese naturopathic medicine as a prostate remedy.

### Cernilton (Standardized Pollen Extract)

Some people use Cernilton to lessen some of the symptoms of BPH, like frequent need for urination and inability to fully empty the bladder. Cernilton is a flower pollen extract and a natural substance derived from flower pollen. Pollen is the male seed of flowers that enables flowering plants to reproduce. People also may benefit from all the wonderful properties of bee pollen.

- Supplies vital nutrients to the body and cells (including all essential amino acids, unsaturated fatty acids and enzymes)
- Improves absorption of vitamins, minerals and trace elements from the food we eat
- Enables better adaptation to stress, enhancing physical and mental capacity

**Helps regulate:**
- Immune system
- Lipid metabolism
- Blood cholesterol level
- Prostate function

**Obignya peciose (babassu)**

This palm tree species is mostly found growing in Brazil. In traditional medicine, it is used to reduce many symptoms of the urinary tract including prostatism.

**Pumpkin seeds**

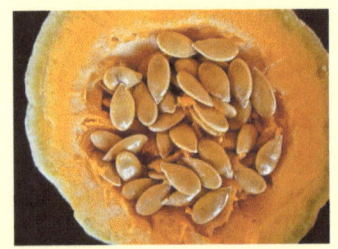

These contain specific kind of sterols. It can improve the flow of urine and augment the emptying of the urinary bladder. Even

10g daily may reduce these problematic symptoms of BPH significantly.

**Urtica**

It contains a lot of antioxidants and antiinflammatory substances. Its features are very similar to palmetto, and that is why both are often used together.

**Lycopene**

Lycopene is a natural pigment present in many fruits and vegetables such as tomatoes. Lycopene can slow the occurrence of BPH symptoms.

The single best source of Lycopene are tomatoes – they also contain a lot of antioxidants, so tomatoes are a good choice. The more pink or red the fruit is, the greater the concentration of lycopene it has. Other Lycopene sources include papaya, grapefruit, watermelon, guava, carrot, red bell pepper, apricot, red cabbage.

**Green tea**

Green tea which contains a lot of antioxidants, bolsters the immunity, and may potentially slow down the development of prostate cancer.

**Zinc**

Dietary supplements containing zinc are a good choice for reducing BPH symptoms. Longlasting shortage of this element may be one of the causes of prostatic disease. Food with good zinc content – poultry, seafood, seeds, nuts, pumpkin are therefore a logical choice.

**Useful prostate care advice:**

- Try to urinate every time before going out of the house.
- Don't drink in the last 2 hours before going to sleep.
- Stay hydrated throughout the day.
- Keep a healthy body weight.
- Exercise consistently.
- Try to avoid stress.
- Avoid products that can cause dehydration e.g. cold medicines.
- Do a prostate medical examination regularly and consult with your doctor if you develop prostate symptoms.

**EXERCISING**

Regular physical activity is always important – so it should not be a surprise, that for prostate health you should aim to consistently exercise.

**Maintain a proper body weight** – this is also really important for prostate health. If you are overweight, increase

the intensity of your daily physical activity while limiting unnecessary caloric intake, and try to lose the extra pounds you may have. This will help you to reduce prostate symptoms.
- Try a mix of cardio, stretching, and strength training.
- Remember to exercise all the muscles groups.
- **More active men develop BPH less often.** Clinical studies confirm that exercising for 5 or more hours a week can decrease the chances of BPH by 30% to even 50%.

Even low or mild intensity activity can suffice in many cases.

Consult with your physician before starting or participating in protracted bicycling exercise. This activity may be not the best choice for men with prostate problems.

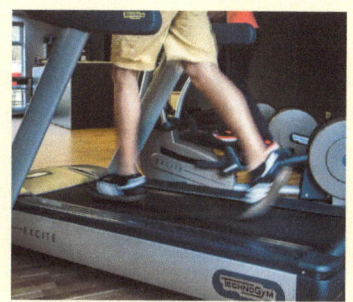

## Kegels

Kegels exercises can be good for you – practice it every day, for a few minutes to bring out the beneficial effects. Kegel exercise can also improve your libido and sexual performance.

The good thing about Kegels exercise is that you can do it wherever and whenever you want irrespective of location or situation. You don't need a special time or day to practice.

## Yoga

Yoga is always a great choice for you. Yoga improves your flexibility and strengthens your muscles. It helps you to relax. Yoga stimulates the blood circulation to all the body parts. It also has many advantages in improving your sexual energy.

## Cardio

Tailored cardiovascular exercise workouts always bring great advantages, no matter what your goals or physical limitations are. You can streng then your body, support your health, and improve your sexual life. As an additional 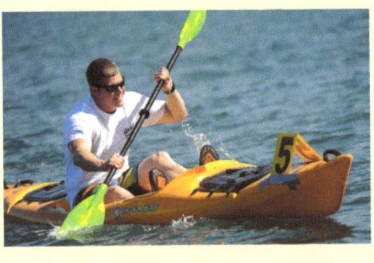 benefit, the blood circulation is improved also– that means longer and better erections, leave alone the cardiovascular health and longevity benefits. **Regular cardiovascular exercise can decrease the chances of erectile dysfunction by 30%.**

## Swimming

Swimming is great not only for muscular strength, but also for libido. Doing this for only 30 minutes a week can really bring about great benefits. Using swimming exercise, one can strengthen the muscles, lose weight, and feel healthier and more attractive. It is an advantage of swimming exercise that it is atraumatic to the joints. Swimming is a favored exercise for those with hip, knee, or spine problems, as the entire body is supported in the water.

# SOURCES

https://heartuk.org.uk/cholesterolanddiet/lowcholesteroldiet-sandfoods
https://www.health.harvard.edu/hearthealth/11foodsthatlowercholesterol
https://www.health.harvard.edu/diabetes/howtoeathealthyawayfromhomeifyouhavediabetes
https://www.health.harvard.edu/blog/healthylifestylecanpreventdiabetesandevenreverseit2018090514698
http://www.diabetes.org/
http://psddrzewica.pl/jaksobieradziczcukrzyca/
www.hsph.harvard.edu/nutritionsource/whatshouldyoueat/
www.nutritionfacts.org/
https://www.poradnikz-drowie.pl/zdrowie/ukladkrwionosny/cwiczeniaktoreobnizazbytwysokiecisnieniekrwiaaxyne8uvHkQxC.html
https://www.menshealth.pl/zdrowie/8sposobownanadcisnienie,4737,1
https://www.webmd.com/hypertensionhighblood-pressure/safeexercisetips#1
https://www.health.harvard.edu/diseasesandconditions/bloodpressurewhatsfoodgottodowithit
https://prostate.net/articles/8greatsexexercisesformen/
https://www.webmd.com/men/features/ex-erciseforprostatehealth
https://www.health.harvard.edu/menshealth/2018annualreportonprostatediseases
https://www.health.harvard.edu/cancer/candiethelp-fightprostatecancer
https://www.health.harvard.edu/stayinghealthy/addsoytoyourdiet-butdontsubtractotherhealthyfoods
https://www.health. harvard.edu/newsletter_article/seleniumandprostatecancer
https://www.health.harvard.edu/press_releases/lifestylechangestotreatprostate
https://www.health.harvard.edu/menshealth/lifestyletherapy-forprostatecancerdoesitwork
https:// www.health.harvard.edu/stayinghealthy/doesy-ourdietdeliver
https://www.health.com/health/gallery/0,,20720182,00.html
http://www.przyprawowy.pl/encyklopediaprzypraw
html https://www.foodmatters.com/article/11herbsthatboostyourbrainpower
https://health.bas-tyr.edu/news/healthtips/2015/02/5hearthealthyherbs
http://naturallysavvy.com/restore/top5herbsfor-fightingfatigue
https://pixabay.com

www.ingramcontent.com/pod-product-compliance
Lightning Source LLC
LaVergne TN
LVHW070048070526
838201LV00036B/353